American Medical Association
Physicians dedicated to the health of America

Cutting Costs in the Physician Practice

Alan S. Whiteman, PhD, FACMPE

Jerry Hermanson, MBA, CHE

Dennis Palkon, PhD, MPH, MSW

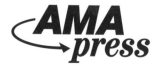

Cutting Costs in the Physician Practice

This book is for information purposes only. It is not intended to constitute legal or financial advice. If legal, financial, or other professional advice is required, the services of a competent professional should be sought.

Additional copies of this book may be ordered by calling 800 621-8335.
Mention product number OP068600

ISBN 1-57947-161-7

BP38:0161-00:3/01

Contents

Preface

Medical practices operate in a dynamic environment that is constantly changing. Due to managed care and reduced reimbursement, physicians face increasing demand for clinical services, placing more and more demand on office staff. In order to manage their practice effectively, physicians must gain significant knowledge in a variety of areas in which they may not have professional training, such as accounting, financial management, purchasing, and human resource management.

The intent of this book is to explain the basic steps that may be followed by a medical practice to reduce operating overhead and enhance productivity for the physician(s) and office staff. Through practical information that may be directly applied to practice operations, this book is designed to be used as a tool to assist physicians in making decisions as they relate to the daily and long-term operations of the medical practice.

Some of the most important decisions a physician makes have long-term implications. Therefore, it is critical that the physician has a strong knowledge base when making major purchases or drastically altering the way a medical practice operates. For example, the physician's position can be strongly enhanced in negotiations by knowing the right questions to ask and being able to properly evaluate the answers received.

The ever-changing healthcare environment also dictates that a physician be able to operate a medical practice like a business. This business must effectively utilize scarce resources and provide quality medical care and outstanding patient service. Only with an understanding of the information provided in this book can a physician begin to develop an information base to make informed and intelligent decisions.

Acknowledgments

The authors would like to thank Mark Kopelman, a senior in Health Administration at Indiana University, for his diligent assistance in researching aspects of this book. We would also like to thank Katharine Dvorak for her timely assistance and helpful effort in ensuring the publication of this manuscript.

About the Authors

Alan S Whiteman, PhD, FACMPE, is both an experienced health care executive and a professor of graduate health administration studies. Dr Whiteman has over 30 years' experience in all facets of the health care industry with over 24 years' experience in managing or consulting with physician practices. In addition, he is the president of Healthcare Integration Consultants, Inc, a professional services firm specializing in assisting physicians in making practices more efficient, effective, and financially sound. He received his PhD from Walden University, his MBA from Wayne State University, and his BA from Michigan State University.

Jerry Hermanson, MBA, CHE, is an experienced health care leader. Mr Hermanson has over 27 years' experience in the industry, including hospital administration, physician organizations, and managed care. Mr Hermanson is chief executive officer of Healthcare Integration Consultants, Inc. In this capacity he provides management and technical services to IPAs, physician practices of all sizes, and medical societies. He is also an adjunct professor of graduate health administration studies. He received his MBA and BSBA from the University of Florida.

Dennis Palkon, PhD, MPH, MSW, is a full professor and past chairman of Health Administration at Florida Atlantic University in Boca Raton, Florida. Dr Palkon has extensive academic and publishing experience. He is also executive editor of *Hospital Topics* and serves on numerous editorial boards. He received his PhD and MPH from the University of Pittsburgh, his MSW from Virginia Commonwealth, and his BS from Villanova University.

Chapter 1

Identifying Areas of Concern

Employing systematic methods to identify a medical practice's expenses and whether the expenses are reasonable is a basic requirement when attempting to contain costs. In addition, an ongoing review of expenses is necessary to ensure continued efforts in cost containment.

There are a number of management tools you can develop to assist you in making such expense determinations. In general, these tools collect data and give you the ability to compare the expenses of your own practice over time or to compare expenses against other practices. Most of these tools are simple in concept and implementation. However, the key to the success of these tools is your ability to accurately identify costs in your practice. If your practice is large, it may already have an accounting system in place that captures the expense data on a regular basis. Such a system can divide practice expenses into categories and can generate regular reports. Smaller groups or solo practices may not have the same accounting capabilities. In these practices it is necessary to work with whoever is providing bookkeeping services and develop a regular method to identify the practices' expenses and separate them into expense categories.

Once an accurate system to identify expenses is in place, you can begin to develop tools to search for cost savings. Areas of concern are usually identified by comparing your practice's costs against internal expectations and external data. It is important to perform both internal and external comparisons to maximize your efforts at cost containment.

Reports of practice expenses must be produced on a monthly basis to be helpful in identifying areas of potential cost savings.

Internal Comparisons

Comparing your actual costs with expected costs requires the development of internal target costs or expenses. This process is known as *budgeting* and is a basic management activity for any size practice.

According to David H. Glusman, CPA, an expense budget is the simplest tool to maintain control over expenses.[1] An expense budget provides a template to identify what you think your expenses should be versus your actual expenses. A difference between your actual expenses and what you budgeted indicates a possible area of cost concern.

Budget Development

Some look at the process of developing a budget as difficult and laborious. But, shared with the key individuals in a practice—including key physicians and managers—the task can be accomplished in a relatively short period of time and may give all participants a new view of how the practice is spending its money.

In developing an expense budget you must first make a list of the various expenses incurred by your practice. This list should include all areas of expenditure except physicians' compensation. In making a list you should refer to your practice's "chart of accounts," which may have been developed by your practice manager or your accountant. This chart of accounts should list all of the expense categories that your accounting system is capturing. It should include areas of general overhead such as rent, telephone expense, utilities, waste removal, and so on. In addition, it should identify various types of supplies used in the practice such as general office supplies, medical supplies, laboratory supplies (if your practice has an in-house lab), or other categories of supplies unique to your practice. This list should also include expenses related to your employees such as salaries, benefit costs, payroll taxes, and other employee-related expenses.

When this list of expense categories has been compiled, the next step is to estimate projected expenditures for each. A good way to begin the process of projecting future expenditures is to compile data organized by expense category from the last several years. By analyzing how your costs have changed over time, you can establish trends that can be the basis of future projections.

Some expense categories will trend based on preestablished formulas and can therefore be estimated with a high degree of accuracy. Expenses such as rent, leases, and other contracted services fall into this type. A review of contracts will give you the basis to establish future cost projections in these expense categories.

Other expenses will trend based on business factors, such as inflation or cost of production. Expenses in this category include most supplies, utility costs, insurance costs, and staff salaries. A percentage increase to these expenses can be established by reviewing projected increases in the consumer price index for medical services and by asking the practice's suppliers if they have projections for future price increases.

In addition, most expenses are affected by the volume of care given in the practice. To factor this in, a percentage increase in service volume must be projected and then applied to those expense categories affected by volume increases before other factors are considered (such as inflation). While some categories of expenses will vary consistently and uniformly with the increase in volume (such as medical supplies, office supplies, and lab supplies), others will occur in steps (such as salaries and equipment costs). Accurately predicting these categories of expenses will be the most difficult.

Budget Comparison

Usually an annual budget that is broken down into monthly projections is developed, as it may be easier to project what the practice's expenditures are on a monthly basis and then compile an annual figure. Whichever method is used, it is important to try and identify how these expenses will fluctuate from month to month. Some expenses will be consistent from month to month, such as rent, while others will change based on volatile factors, such as volume of care given (ie, supplies). Still others will vary based on payment schedules, such as employee taxes and other insurance expenses. A review of historic expenditures will give a good indication of which categories will change from month to month and which will be consistent.

Once an expense budget is finalized it can become a powerful tool to identify where the practice is incurring its costs. To effectively utilize an expense budget, however, actual expenditures must be reviewed on at least a monthly basis. Variations between actual and projected spending should be carefully researched to determine the cause of the variation and whether there is need to make any changes affecting the expenditures.

While the practice manager should make the initial review of the monthly expense report and research explanations for any variances discovered, the practice's managing physician must do the final review. If effective cost containment is to be accomplished, the physician must take a leadership role and be directly involved in the budgeting process on a regular basis. Such involvement does not have to be time-consuming, but it must be consistent. Review of the expense budget performance can be made a regular part of your monthly management meeting with your key office staff and physician group, for example.

Payroll Reports

While salary expenses are part of your overall expense budget, you will need to develop an additional report to properly review these expenses. A *payroll report* comparing actual hours worked to budgeted hours helps to identify excessive costs.

Practices that have part-time employees must have a report that compares actual hours worked with budgeted hours. A simple look at overtime will not readily identify excess hours worked by part-time employees, as excess hours will not generate overtime situations unless the employee works more than 40 hours during a given week. Therefore, a report listing each employee's scheduled hours and actual hours worked should be generated for each pay period. This report can be reviewed monthly with the general expense budget comparisons.

When looking at a payroll report, it is important to look at regular hours worked as well as overtime hours.

Included in the payroll report should be a list, by employee, of all overtime paid. As overtime is usually paid on a time-and-a-half basis, a reduction or elimination of any overtime is key for cost containment. If you are routinely scheduling overtime because the practice's patient volume is growing, careful, ongoing analysis should be undertaken to determine when it is financially beneficial to hire new employees who can be paid for regular hours.

Most formal in-house payroll systems and all outside payroll service companies can provide payroll reports on a routine basis. Again, review them at least monthly.

External Comparisons

Comparing your practice's expenses or performance to outside indicators is another source of identifying areas of potential cost containment. This process is sometimes referred to as *benchmarking*. According to Joan M. Roediger, JD, LLM, benchmarking provides a more structured approach to establishing business parameters and reviewing financial progress against baseline values.[2]

Physician practices can take advantage of these techniques by obtaining benchmark data from outside sources and comparing the data against their performance. Most outside benchmarks are based on surveys of other medical practices in the same geographic area as your practice as well as nationwide.

Sources of Benchmark Data

There are numerous organizations that collect data that can be used for comparison against your practice. These sources include the American Medical Association, numerous health care magazines, professional and specialty societies for both physicians and health care consultants, and various local organizations. In addition, a careful review of medical publications can yield a wealth of sources from surveys that are available for the asking.

Many of these sources look at a very limited set of data. Others, such as the Medical Group Management Association's (MGMA) annual survey of physician group practices, provide data for numerous expense and revenue categories based on geographic region, medical specialty, group size, and several other parameters.

It is also possible to develop local or regional data through surveys you and your colleagues may agree to develop and compile. This can be particularly helpful if your area is unique due to local factors. For example, data such as salary costs can vary greatly over larger geographic areas, so local surveys may be the best source of good comparative data. Consider asking your county medical society to help develop benchmark data.

Validation of Benchmark Data

Before you compare benchmark data against your practice, you must understand the method used to solicit the data as well as the definitions used in the surveys. The data gathered may not be directly comparable to your practice's data, or you may need to recalculate your practice's data in order to compare it against the benchmark data. Data that are given for large geographic areas may not be meaningful for your particular area, for example. Rural and urban data, likewise, may not be comparable.

Data that are collected for specific specialty practices is generally better for comparison. However, try to determine what services or procedures are included in the practices surveyed, as that may have a significant effect on the comparability of the data to your practice.

Benchmark Data on Practice Expenses

For purposes of cost containment, only benchmark data on expenses are relevant. You may, however, wish to look at other types of data with which to compare your practice, such as revenue and productivity data. Revenue and compensation data are always important to physicians and are natural categories to review at least on a yearly basis. These comparisons are particularly important when considering the addition of a new physician or physician extender to a practice. (See Chapter 6 for information on recruiting additional practitioners.)

Overhead generally runs between 55% and 65% of total revenue.[3] This excludes compensation paid to physicians. As a result, significant savings can result in higher compensation to physicians. Therefore, a comparison of your practice's overhead to national and regional data for your specialty is a key expenses factor to benchmark.

Data on the various components of the practice's overhead can also be compared. The number of personnel per physician is another key comparison, as salary costs can run as high as 50% of the overhead of a practice. In addition, salaries for each category of employee are an important item to compare—in tight labor markets, low salaries can make it difficult to attract and retain good employees.

Other data categories include virtually all other expense categories for which you can receive data. The more you compare, the better a picture you get of your practice in relation to others.

Analysis of External Data

External data that represent overall practice performance, such as total overhead as a percent of revenue, should be compared on an annual basis. Monthly data or other periods of less than a year may be affected by seasonal fluctuations in your practice's expenses. Even individual expense category data are not comparable over short periods.

Data that identify categories that do not change much with time can be compared on a one-shot basis. Salary levels are an example of data that are comparable with your current figures. Other examples include annual malpractice premiums, other annual insurance premiums, and individual supply items.

Guidelines for Comparing Data

Once the comparative data have been validated to your satisfaction, variations from your performance against the benchmark data will begin to be of value. However, it is important to fully research any significant differences between your practice's data and the internal or external data.

Unique factors within your practice must be considered before a final determination is made as to whether your costs are reasonable. Often, budget comparisons, particularly in the first year or two, will show variations due to inaccurate budgeting. Your budgeting accuracy will improve with time.

Carefully validate the data you are using and make comparisons of similar expense categories for the most accurate time period. Developing a handful of reports that you regularly review will give you the tools needed to identify potential cost savings for your practice. It can also give you better knowledge with which you can oversee your practice.

External data usually represent general averages or ranges of expenses collected by a single or specific survey. Averages may not be good indicators if the response to the survey was low. A good survey will indicate the percentage of responses or give other data that will help you decide if the figures are worth using. In addition, external data that are developed from multiple specialty practices may not yield comparable data for your specialty.

Endnotes

1. Glusman DH. Benchmarking physician practice expenses. *Physician's News Digest.* May 1999.

2. Roediger JM. Formally benchmarking your medical practice. *Physician's News Digest.* August 1999.

3. Kostreski F, ed. Managing your practice to lower overhead. *Pediatric News.* 1997.

Chapter 2

Work Smarter, Not Harder! A Systems Approach

*D*r Brown entered his office at 9:15 AM after completing two complex hospital visits. The lobby was filled with patients and the staff was scrambling to deal with the morning's myriad of problems. Because of the health care industry changes that had occurred in recent years, such as the increase in managed care and numerous regulatory requirements placed on practices, the staff continuously "plugged holes in the dike" to get the various required tasks completed and have the patients see Dr Brown. Unfortunately, because of increased workloads, high turnover, and confusing and cumbersome rules and regulations, the practice was in chaos and the staff demoralized.

Many physician practices have experienced an increase in both patient and paperwork loads, an increase in demand for physician and staff time, and a reduction in revenue. These factors have been greatly exaggerated by the fact that many medical offices evolved without formal planning or design. Thus, when more demands are made on an already taxed system, the system collapses.

If Dr Brown's scenario sounds familiar, it is time to look at the potential benefits of re-engineering and process improvement. *Re-engineering* is the task of reviewing the practice operation and finding a simpler and more efficient method to complete all of the tasks involved in operating the practice. *Process improvement* entails reviewing each procedure and methodology that is used and finding a more effective and less labor-intensive way to complete that task.

In today's office environment, the mention of re-engineering often causes an immediate reaction to begin automating all office functions. While automation is an option, focusing strictly on automation becomes too narrow a scope. (Examples of automated systems include patient scheduling and accounts receivable management. Manual systems might include such functions as patient flow in the practice or telephone communications.)

There is a definite need for a combination of automated and manual systems that interface to fulfill the needs of the medical practice. This chapter discusses how to review your practice, how to review both types of systems at work in your practice, and how, if properly designed and utilized, these systems can reduce physician downtime and reduce staff stress.

Reviewing Your Practice

The only means to improve your practice's operations is to review and revise the systems that are currently in place. Thus, the first step in reviewing, or re-engineering, your practice is to thoroughly examine and record each step that is taken in the completion of various tasks.

The most effective way to record a procedure is to either write a brief step-by-step summary or sketch out the workflow in a diagram. It is extremely important for the individual reviewing the work process to understand the nuances of the specific tasks being studied. Make sure that you repeatedly ask the individual who performs each task to go over each step and to not leave out any details. Once the procedures are documented, observe the individuals performing the tasks on several occasions to ensure that you have not missed a key step in your documentation.

A key question to ask your employees or your office manager is how a specific procedure evolved. This question should be followed by further questions, asking why this procedure is followed and how long it has been performed in this manner.

Manual Systems

The financial success of a medical practice is completely dependent on physician productivity, which is driven by efficiently and effectively seeing patients and performing procedures day after day. By optimizing physician productivity, the practice also increases patient satisfaction and enhances referral opportunities. Thus, the strategic areas in your practice that will benefit the most from re-engineering and process improvement pertain to patient-related processes. These include the following manual systems: telephone communications, patient scheduling, and practice flow.

The best place to start an assessment of practice systems is at the practice's initial point of contact with a patient: the telephone call received from a patient. This initial contact with the patient, the information exchanged, and processing the information are the first steps in a manual process that have a critical impact on the practice operations and the cost of operating the practice. Effective and efficient systems reduce operating overhead and constantly play a key role in containing costs, which ultimately can lead to increased revenues.

Keep Staff Involved

It is important to remember that the most complex part of making changes in a business entity, particularly in a medical practice, is gaining the full support and cooperation of your staff. Employees who do not understand the sudden desire to change "the way things have always been done" may resist the change and can defeat the re-engineering process. Therefore, it is imperative that, prior to beginning the re-engineering process, you communicate your goals and objectives to your staff, solicit their support, and explain the direct benefits to them. Remember, consistent two-way communication with your employees is the key to your success!

Telephone Communications   During an initial review of the telephone system, it is important to separate the electronic communication system from the manual aspects of human intervention. The key to successful evaluation of the telephone communication system is to evaluate the following:

1. **Greeting of the caller.** The staff person answering the telephone should establish the caller's identity.

2. **Triage of the call.** Is the call a medical issue? Billing issue? If the caller is a patient, does he or she want to make an appointment? Need directions? Or is it a nonmedical call?

3. **Length of initial call.** Does the staff person greet the caller, triage the call, and satisfy the caller's needs in a reasonable amount of time?

Experienced employees should be able to effectively greet a caller, triage the call, and meet the caller's initial needs in less than one minute. If calls are taking longer on a regular basis, then the employee is not judiciously managing his or her time. Employees answering the telephones should have a standardized script that they use on all calls. This script can be modified to adapt to callers they know or to deal with unusual circumstances.

Managing the telephone process properly will alleviate one of the biggest bottlenecks in patient flow that occurs in a medical office. Automated telephone attendants and other electronic systems can enhance and improve a good manual system, but they are only a stopgap measure if a good flow and system are not in place.

Upon completion of the review of the telephone answering process, it is important to review each problem or bottleneck, prepare a solution for the problem, and teach the employees the proper method of handling each situation. Role-playing, if properly utilized, is a tool that can be used at a staff meeting to teach proper telephone technique. A sound telephone response system can also reduce stress and the need to hire additional personnel.

Patient Scheduling   Once the telephone communications system has been reviewed and the office staff trained on the proper use of the system, scheduling patient visits is the next critical area to review. A good scheduling system can increase physician productivity, increase practice revenue, and help contain labor costs.

Stop thinking in blocks of 10, 15, 20, and 30 minutes. Instead, look at the system as scheduling for the specific problem. Some patients may only need a few minutes with the doctor, for example, and most visits could be categorized into *short, medium,* or *long.*[2]

Increased patient flow does not mean less patient service.[1] *Therefore, during the scheduling review process, throw out preconceived concepts and look for new ways to enhance the process.*

The key element to scheduling goes back to the quality of the initial telephone communication: finding out what the patient needs when the appointment is scheduled. Experience with the practice will enable you to determine how many visits of each category appear in the practice each day.

Once the current patient scheduling system has been reviewed and revisions are proposed, prepare a written procedure that explains in detail the process to be followed. To ensure that the procedure will work, review the proposed process with your staff, get their input, and fine-tune the procedure. After the procedure is implemented, periodically review the process and make sure it is being followed. Changing behavior is a difficult and complex process. If the changes are not monitored continuously, individuals may revert to old behavior.

Upon the successful implementation of new scheduling procedures, the practice can begin the process of using an electronic scheduling system. Remember, automation is not a substitute for good procedures—it is just a means of enhancing and streamlining a good work process.

Practice Flow   One of the basics of efficient and effective office operation is the patient and staff traffic flow as they move through the office all day long. This traffic flow has significant ramifications on the entire practice. The traffic pattern in the practice determines the number of staff members with patient contact and the number of employees required to process the patients. If you reduce the number of staff necessary for regular face-to-face patient contact, you can reduce the office traffic and possibly the number of employees.[3]

Many practices have employees literally tripping over each other and the patients. Why? Because no one has defined their job responsibilities or provided a defined workstation for their duties. It is important that employees have job descriptions that explain their roles and responsibilities.

It is also critical that, as the practice is being reviewed, the patient flow is tracked for a period of time to learn exactly how and why a patient is managed in a specific way. One must define all of the steps to determine if parts of the process are unnecessary, are duplicated by the physician, or have simply "always been done this way." Remember, if the patient is not in the room waiting for the doctor, the practice has just increased inefficiency and decreased physician productivity.

During the review process, carefully observe the check-in and check-out areas of the practice. It is important to make sure that there is enough space during peak periods to handle the volume of patients requiring assistance. During this observation, make sure that your staffing patterns enable adequate staff to support each function during peak periods.

In many cases, the physician is a key contributor to traffic interruptions in the practice. Most doctors have good work habits and stay focused on patient care during office hours. But, in some instances, the staff, through poor communication about office procedures, disrupts the traffic flow by taking the doctor out of production. It is imperative that once the doctor begins seeing patients he or she is not interrupted (except for urgent patient care issues or for specific reasons the doctor has communicated to the staff).

Office Layout In the process of reviewing manual systems in the practice, it is important to also look at the physical layout of the practice site. The practice site was, most likely, established at the onset of your practice, and in many cases, the practice has evolved into something different. Undoubtedly, the volume of patients has increased significantly. Unless the review determines that the practice site is too small or will not meet future practice demands, the most expedient activity is to enhance the practice through the review and modification process.

Patient Education Reviewing the manual systems and implementing effective procedures is only half of the battle. The other half of the battle is educating patients on office policy and procedure. This is a crucial step if practice economies and effectiveness are to be accomplished.

Educating patients is accomplished through a combination of methods. First, the practice should instruct the patient on office policy each time he or she calls the office. Staff may tell the patient that he or she must arrive 15 minutes early to complete paperwork or that he or she must bring a specimen, and so on. This must be reinforced at the visit by the staff reminding the patients of their responsibilities. In addition, the office should provide written literature in the lobby and in the exam rooms regarding the procedures the patients must follow.

Electronic Systems

Once the practice has completed its fine-tuning of the manual systems it uses throughout its daily operation, it is time to focus on the practice's automated systems.

Cost Containment

Our goal is to contain cost and reduce overhead—not to look for increasing expenses.

During the entire review process our energies have been focused on streamlining the office and improving the practice's manual systems. The key benefit of this process is to maximize the utilization of office personnel. Human resources are the most costly element in your practice. Thus, it is critical that you use this resource effectively and conserve it. If the practice is properly reviewed and modified, problems will be solved and additional staff will not be hired unnecessarily. It is key to remember: "Never hire staff to plug holes in the dike."

The time invested in reviewing your practice will have long-term benefits. "Improving or altering each step in the patient flow process can produce long-lasting results in patient satisfaction and in maximizing revenues."[4] Remember, if you review your operations and find that everything is working well, leave it alone. Keep the adage "If it isn't broke, don't fix it" in mind.

Defining System Needs It is important to reflect on the practices' needs before immediately selecting the automated systems to implement. In today's managed care environment, medical practices require a great deal of sophisticated information to properly manage operations. Thus, the search for a new system should encompass looking for the information required to manage the medical practice.

The most common approach to selecting a new system is to identify the weaknesses in the current system and try to fill in these gaps. The problem with this approach, however, is that the practice can miss valuable opportunities to revamp or enhance present operations if it is simply looking for stopgaps to fix inadequacies in the current system.

The information that the practice should have readily available in its information system can be defined in two broad categories (the reports listed here are a sample of the options available):

1. **Financial Accounting Reports.** These include:
   - *Accounts payable*: a listing of expenses that have been paid
   - *Balance sheet*: a statement of practice assets and liabilities
   - *Income and expense statements*: a report of revenue and expenses for the current period and a comparison of a previous period

2. **Managerial Accounting Reports.** These include:
   - *Accounts receivable management reports:*
     a. Aged analysis of accounts receivable
     b. Aged analysis of accounts receivable by payor
     c. Procedure analysis by the CPT® medical code and order of volume
     d. Diagnosis analysis
     e. Production report by doctor and/or other provider
     f. Referring physician analysis
     g. Miscellaneous reports designed for the practice and a report generator
     h. Scheduling reports, including:
        - Patient lag time between call and appointment
        - No-show report
        - Appointment reminder calls
        - Office waiting time between arrival and visit
     i. Demographic reports on patients
     j. Managed care reports for contract management, including:
        - Utilization report: charges to collections
        - Cost of providing services
        - Capitation profitability

Selection Process   Typically, computer systems in medical practices were selected for a single purpose: billing. Unfortunately, today's health care environment dictates more sophisticated requirements for the medical practice than an electronic billing system that simply prints claims forms and may or may not transmit electronic insurance claims. To successfully manage a medical practice in the current health care environment, it is necessary for a practice to have a versatile practice management system.

Modern technology has significantly improved practice management information systems over the past few years to meet the demands of managed care and other changes in the industry. The wide acceptance of patient scheduling, electronic claims submission, and increased interest and demand for electronic medical records have pushed software vendors to make major strides in their offerings. This factor, coupled with advances in hardware and reduction in cost, has fueled major changes in the products on the market.

The first step in determining the information system needs for your practice is to jot down the critical goals you want to accomplish with an electronic system. Following are a few sample goals that the practice may wish to expand upon:

1. Select a leading vendor that will still be in business in 5 years.

2. Include functional areas for the changing industry (ie, managed care, electronic medical records, office scheduling).

3. Establish a realistic timeline.

4. Implement a rough budget.

The second step is to develop a document that can be used as a *request for information* (RFI) and/or a *request for proposal* (RFP). The purpose of this document is to collect consistent data that can be compared for decision-making.

It is of paramount importance that the office staff is involved in this process and that they are encouraged to include elements that would not only enhance their work but also complement the manual systems that currently exist in the medical practice. The document should be created in sections that focus on specific aspects of the practice. A document of this nature not only is important in obtaining quotes but also focuses everyone's attention during system demonstrations.

Once the document is created, the practice should select several practice management system vendors and contact their marketing representatives. (See Appendix A for a list of the leading health care system vendors in the marketplace today.) The practice should share the selection document with the vendors to ensure that their systems can meet your requirements. Those that can should be invited to demonstrate their product to the office staff. The number of vendors selected should be limited to three to five or the process can become cumbersome, time-consuming, and ineffective.

A demonstration should be established at the practice site for each of the selected vendors. Each member of the office staff should have a copy of the selection document and should independently evaluate each of the systems that are reviewed. Upon completion of the review process, all of the staff evaluations should be reviewed and tabulated. The vendors whose systems meet all or the majority of the criteria should then have an opportunity to bid on the system.

As a part of the final review process, each vendor should be requested to supply a list of references. It is imperative that these references be contacted without the marketing representative present. The individual making the reference calls should have a specific list of questions. And, if possible, he or she should visit the office of reference to speak with the staff members using the system. In addition, the office staff member conducting this process should review the system manuals that are provided by the vendor to see if they are easy to use and understand.

It is critical to remember that an electronic system must fit the practice, not vice versa. Do not allow marketing representatives to sell you something that resembles placing a square peg in a round hole.

If all of the systems reviewed have similar pricing and features, the review then needs to go to the next level. The reviewer must have a second checklist in order to ask consistent questions for comparison. These questions should focus on system downtime, telephone support availability, support response time to calls, and other questions or concerns. (Appendix B contains a sample selection evaluation form to use when choosing between various physician practice management systems.)

After the completion of a thorough review process, the practice should have eliminated some of the competitors in the process. It is suggested that the process lead to two finalists in the bidding competition. In "Selecting Practice Management Information Systems," Robin Worley and Vincent Ciotti suggest that both of the finalists in the process be aware of the competitive bidding to afford the practice strong negotiating clout.[5] The authors further state:

- Involving end users heavily in evaluating systems not only gains their detailed input on features but also increases their "buy in;"

- Structured checklists can make steps such as telephone references and site visits as quantifiable as any RFP score;

- Perusing user manuals not only avoids marketing hyperbole but also serves as an excellent product definition for the contract; and

- Keeping two vendors in the running at the end, rather than having a single RFP winner, greatly increases negotiating clout.

Taking Bold New Steps

The business world has rapidly advanced into an environment rich in electronic technology, yet the business side of medicine has not kept pace. A quantum leap for medical practices is to implement and utilize electronic medical records. This can be an exciting, yet challenging, change.

Electronic Medical Records

Practice efficiencies can be greatly enhanced through the implementation of an electronic medical record system. In "Choosing and Implementing a Reliable Electronic Patient Record System," Patty Edwards-Capella states, "To gain the full benefits of an EPR [enterprise-wide patient record] system, it is important to first ensure efficient and cost-effective work processes are in place."[6] Thus, an electronic medical record system can only be instituted and used effectively if the practice has been reviewed and modified to enhance operations.

The use of an electronic medical record system can also bring tangible, intangible, and nonfinancial benefits to the practice. Table 2.1 lists the benefits of electronic medical records systems as summarized in the article, "Cost Justifying Electronic Medical Records."[7]

Table 2.1: Sample Benefits of Electronic Medical
Records Systems

	Tangible Financial Benefits	Intangible Financial Benefits	Nonfinancial Benefits
Product Enhancement	• Reduction in chart pulls reduces labor cost in medical records department • Automated interfaces reduce labor costs for personnel involved in coding, billing, manually retrieving lab results, and referral coordination • Transcription costs • Malpractice premium lowered • Less dictation time, faster documentation of encounters • Improved charge capture, documenting home health management • Reduced nurse intake time • Faster billing reduces cash cycle, cuts receivable days • Document storage space costs reduced	• Scheduling of resources becomes more efficient • Easier QA and UR reporting • Less time spent copying, filing, faxing, and transmitting data • Lower supply costs • Fewer lab results lost, fewer repeat tests • Aggregate patient data improves financial forecasting, risk assumption • Automation of referral process and more appropriate use of specialists	
Quality of Care Improvements	• Automated protocols/guidelines reduce expensive variations in patient treatment • Less time needed to search through records for relevant patient information • Decrease in lost lab reports reduces cost of repeat lab tests	• Reduced medication errors, adverse drug interactions • Improved primary and preventive care (through automated reminders, protocols, and alerts) reduces disease management costs, specialty, and inpatient care • Availability of chart vastly improved • Improved data analysis, outcomes measurement, population-based care • Remote access to patient charts • Summary screen helps prevent overlooked patient information • Ease of providing summary information helps specialists with care	• Improved quality of documentation • Improved outcomes reporting • Less information falls through the cracks in a continuum of care

	Tangible Financial Benefits	Intangible Financial Benefits	Nonfinancial Benefits
Improved Customer Service Satisfaction		• Less need for repeat lab testing • Ease of getting medication refills authorized; faster turnaround time on refill requests • Less paperwork as patients move throughout the health care system	• Confidence physicians are using the best information technology available • Improved communication with preformatted letters, educational handouts, etc.
Increased Professional Satisfaction	• More time to spend with patients	• Reduction in paperwork • Improved communication and less time consumed with routine information exchange	• Increased satisfaction with availability, documentation of records, efficiency of chart reviews and signing, etc. • Ease of covering for other providers' patients • Ease of tracking referred patients

Electronic medical records are a newer innovation when compared to other aspects of practice management systems. Making the correct choice for the practice will have significant long-range implications.

For example, some electronic medical record systems are now available online at a nominal cost. The online systems carry with them a concern for confidentiality and security of critical medical records information; however, it is apparent that some of these systems have an excellent security system and are worthy of consideration. Online systems bring with them a significant cost savings and require no major capital outlays to become operational.

In "Choosing and Implementing a Reliable Electronic Patient Record System," Patty Edwards-Capella offers the following 10 guidelines to follow when choosing an electronic medical records system, which are of paramount importance in planning and implementing an electronic medical records system that will be both productive and cost-effective[8]:

1. **Process Improvement.** For an electronic medical record system to function effectively, the practice must have accomplished all of the

requisite tasks and changes required from the re-engineering and process improvement discussed earlier in this chapter.

2. **Full On-Site Planning and Implementation Support.** Vendor selection is critical to the success of the project. After a careful planning process is completed, the process will require ongoing competent technical support.

3. **Modular, Scalable Design**. The implementation process should be gradual and eventually cover the entire practice. By being modular, the system you select will enable this type of growth process.

4. **Open, Nonproprietary Architecture**. The system should be based on industry standards and enable easy integration with various information systems.

5. **Customizable Workflow**. The system must have the capability to be modified to accommodate the practice workflow.

6. **Customizable Security**. Pick a system that enables the user to modify security and limit access to various applications.

7. **Electronic Data and Scanned Document Support.** The system must have the capability of incorporating both paper-originated and electronic data.

8. **Remote Access/Physician Office Integration**. The system should provide access to remote users.

9. **Health Care Dedication/Proven Record.** Follow the process earlier in this chapter regarding making reference checks.

10. **Applications to Improve Efficiency.** Ideally the system will contain applications designed to automate specific work processes and improve efficiencies, therefore aiding in cost containment.

The electronic medical record system, as a component of the practice management system, must interface with all of your other electronic systems in your practice. The system must work within the constraints of the practice and must complement the manual systems that are currently in place. The system, if utilized properly, can reduce costs, increase physician productivity, and enhance quality of patient care. Table 2.2 offers a list of several practice management software companies.

Table 2.2: Practice Management Software Companies

Company	Contact Information
Companion Technologies	800 717-2517
Nuesoft Technologies	800 453-2702
InfoSys	888 463-6797
PCN (Physician Computer Network)	973 490-3100
Medic Computer Systems	800 334-8534
SCINET Medical Management Systems	800 989-3445
Medical Manager	800 222-7701
MediSoft	800 333-4747
Visionary Medical Systems	888 895-2466

Medical Economics, May 1999

Electing to convert to an electronic medical record system has some significant financial implications. The best method to review the costs and savings of an electronic medical record system is to develop a simple worksheet that lists the cash outlays for the new system and the cost savings that will be gained over a period of time. It is important to understand that implementing a new system will not have an immediate reduction in overhead, but that over a period of time the practice will gain this benefit.

Following is a worksheet that can be used to calculate the overall cost and savings of the system. (This is a step that can be delegated to an office manager.)

Cost Savings Analysis for Electronic Medical Records

Expenditure

Hardware   _____

Software   _____

Estimated 5-year cost   _____

Cost Reduction

Staff reduction   _____

    File clerk   _____

    Transcriptionist   _____

Supplies no longer needed   _____

Estimated 5-year saving   _____

Increased Physician Productivity

(Number of additional encounters
× average revenue) × 5 years   _____

Net Financial Gain to Practice

Expenditure   _____

Less Cost Reduction   _____

    Sub-total   _____

    Plus increased production   _____

Automated Telephone Systems

Earlier in this chapter we discussed automated telephone systems. Many people have a negative reaction to placing a telephone call and having it answered by an automated attendant. But, from a management perspective, it can be a great asset to the practice and the patients. A system that is properly designed and managed can prevent frustrating busy signals for patients, properly direct the calls to the most appropriate individual, and allocate work loads to the entire office staff.

The simplest approach to selecting the appropriate automated telephone system for your office is to find the right vendor for your needs. The selected vendor should be presented with an RFP that lists all of your current needs and anticipated future growth. If the practice is not comfortable with this approach, one or more vendors should be asked to conduct a *needs analysis* of the practice and make recommendations with regard to one or more appropriate systems. Remember, as with anything else you purchase, a vendor will try to sell its best product with all the "bells and whistles." In most instances, the practice will not require all the sophisticated add-ons to the system. All the practice needs is a system that meets your basic needs to provide service to your patients and an effective tool for your staff.

What Makes It Work?

Two-way communication is the basic building block of sound management practices. Always tell your employees what you are trying to accomplish and how they will be a part of this change. The employees may have excellent ideas for modifying manual systems and about application issues for a new practice management information system.

How does a practice make all these changes and make them work? The most basic element of successfully managing the change process is to make all of the practice employees a part of the process. Meaningful involvement in re-engineering and process improvement builds a team that develops consensus and ownership in the changes that evolve. Many people are fearful of changes in their environment because something new can create anxiety and concern. Therefore, encouraging and insisting on participation in the development and implementation of changes help makes employees better understand the reason for change and encourage them to offer input and insight.

As the practice creates or modifies new manual systems, it is imperative that step-by-step procedures be documented for the new system. These procedures are necessary for training the staff and ensuring that each new employee who joins the practice will follow the same protocol. It is of critical importance that, as the manual systems are finalized, the practice constantly trains, retrains, and reassess. Never assume that everyone understands the procedure and how it is to be followed.

Endnotes

1. Conomikes G. *Conomikes Report on Medical Practice Management and Managed Care*. 18(1):4, 5; 98.

2. Conomikes G. *Conomikes Report on Medical Practice Management and Managed Care*. 18(1):4, 5; 98.

3. Boden TW. Study office flow patterns to avoid bottlenecks in your new design. *Physician's Advisory*. February 2000;(2):9, 10.

4. Dunevitz B. Maximize resources by re-engineering your medical group's patient flow process. MGM *Update*. February 15, 2000;39(4):1, 6.

5. Worley R, Ciotti V. Selecting practice management information systems. MGM *Journal*. May/June 1997;44(3):55-56, 58, 60, 62, 64-65, 78.

6. Edwards-Capella P. Choosing and implementing a reliable electronic patient record system. *Healthcare Informatics*. March 1998;15(3, Suppl): 3-5.

7. Renner K. Cost justifying electronic medical records. *Healthcare Financial Management*. October 1996.

8. Edwards-Capella P. Choosing and implementing a reliable electronic patient record system. *Healthcare Informatics*. March, 1998;15(3, Suppl): 3-5.

Chapter 3

Getting the Right People for the Job

One of the most important factors in ensuring success for physician practices is the recruitment and retention of good employees. *Good employees* are associates who can help create a positive work culture, help provide quality health care, and help to contain costs.

Recruiting "Good" Employees

In *Human Resource Management: An Experiential Approach*, John Bernardin and Joyce Russell note that real-world organizational staffing is replete with examples of ineffective and/or inferior methods of recruiting personnel.[1] One of the best ways for physicians to contain costs is to pay special attention to recruiting and retaining personnel who fit best within their work culture.

Determining the Work Culture

Before the recruitment process can begin, physicians must first determine what type of work culture they hope to establish and understand their own values and the values of those they are seeking to employ. To help in this determination, physicians may wish to consult and/or use standardized tools. For example, one appropriate tool is Rudolf Moos' Work Environment Scale, which consists of 90 true and false statements in addition to an assessment of 10 "environmental dimensions" such as involvement, peer cohesion, supervisor support, autonomy, task orientation, and work pressure.[2]

Another helpful tool is Milton Rokeach's Value Survey, which has the respondent rank in order 18 instrumental and 18 terminal values.[3] Rokeach's Value Survey could be used when attempting to assess whether potential employees possess values desired in the physician's practice. The survey could also be used in interviews whereby the applicant could expand on his or her answers in the interview.

Establishing Job Descriptions

It is best to establish job descriptions that delineate what jobs, activities, behaviors, and duties are expected of an employee. Bernardin and Russell note that identifying the critical knowledge abilities, skills, and other characteristics (or KASOCs) is crucial when developing job descriptions, as these job descriptions will assist physicians and/or medical office managers in determining how the work gets completed and by whom.

Methods of Recruitment

Once the physician practice identifies jobs that need to be filled, the recruitment process begins. Some of the more common methods for recruiting personnel include newspaper advertising; visits to high schools, community colleges, and universities; notices to professional associations; referrals; and posting job positions to the Internet.

Job advertisements should always specify the minimum educational and experience requirements. Once a pool of candidates is identified, physician practices should have potential employees complete an application and any other appropriate information release forms. (See the following sidebars for a sample application for employment and a sample disclosure statement and release form.) It is also suggested that reference and/or background checks, as well as perhaps a standardized test and a structural interview, be required of all finalists.

Assistance in creating job descriptions can be obtained from colleagues, consultants, national training and certifying organizations, and various manuals such as David Jay's, The Essential Personnel Sourcebook[4] *and W. R. Lawsons'* How To Develop a Personnel Policy Manual.[5]

Sample Application for Employment

To the applicant: *[Practice Name]* is an equal opportunity employer and complies with all applicable federal, state, and local laws. No question on this application is used for the purpose of limiting or excusing any applicant from consideration for employment on a basis prohibited by local, state, or federal law.

PLEASE PRINT

Position(s) applied for _____ Date of application _____

Name _____ Social Security # _____

Address _____

City _____ State _____ Zip _____

Telephone # _____ Other phone # _____

Are you 18 years of age or older?   _____ Yes _____ No
(If under 18, applicant will be required to submit a birth certificate or work
certificate as required by state and/or federal law.)

Have you ever been terminated for other   _____ Yes _____ No
than economic reasons?

If yes, please explain _____

Have you ever been convicted of, or pleaded guilty or _____ Yes _____ No
no contest to, a crime in the last seven (7) years?

If yes, please explain _____

Do you have the legal right to work in the   _____ Yes _____ No
United States?
(Successful applicants will be required to prove identity and eligibility of
employment.)

Driver's license number if driving is an essential job function:

_____ State: _____

Type of employment desired: Full-time _____ Part-time _____

Date available _____

SKILLS AND QUALIFICATIONS

Summarize any training, skills, licenses, and/or certificates that may qualify you for the job for which you are applying.

_____

_____

_____

_____

EDUCATIONAL BACKGROUND

Proof of education and training may be required upon employment.

Name and Location	Years Completed	Did you graduate?	
High School/GED			Course of Study
_____	_____	___ Yes ___ No	_____
College or University			Major/Degree
_____	_____	___ Yes ___ No	_____
Additional Schooling			Major/Degree
_____	_____	___ Yes ___ No	_____

EMPLOYMENT HISTORY

Provide the following information for your past four (4) employers, assignments, or volunteer activities, starting with the most recent.

From	To	Employer	Telephone
Job Title		Address	
Immediate Supervisor and Title		Summarize the nature of work performed and job responsibilities	
Reason for leaving			
Hourly Rate/Salary		Start $ per Final $ per	

From   To   Employer   Telephone

Job Title   Address

Immediate Supervisor and Title   Summarize the nature of work performed and
                                              job responsibilities

Reason for leaving

Hourly Rate/Salary   Start $ per   Final $ per

From   To   Employer   Telephone

Job Title   Address

Immediate Supervisor and Title   Summarize the nature of work performed and
                                              job responsibilities

Reason for leaving

Hourly Rate/Salary   Start $ per   Final $ per

From   To   Employer   Telephone

Job Title   Address

Immediate Supervisor and Title   Summarize the nature of work performed and
                                              job responsibilities

Reason for leaving

Hourly Rate/Salary   Start $ per   Final $ per

REFERENCES

Please give the name of three persons not related to you, whom you have known for at least one year.

Name	Address	Years Known	Telephone #
1.			
2.			
3.			

EMPLOYMENT APPLICATION CERTIFICATION

I certify that this application was completed by me. I certify that the information in my application, in my resume, and in my interviews is true, complete, and correct. I understand that falsification or omission, whenever or however discovered, may jeopardize my opportunities for employment or, if hired, may be reason for termination of employment. While this application will be given every consideration, its receipt does not imply or guarantee that I will be employed.

If hired, in consideration of my employment, I agree to adhere to the policies and procedures of [Practice Name]. I understand that employment is for an indefinite duration and is terminable at will by either [Practice Name] or myself and that this application does not constitute a contract of employment.

I also understand and agree that the at-will nature of this employment can only be modified by written agreement between parties. I understand that no manager or representative other than the President/CEO (or assigned designee) has any authority to enter into any agreement for employment for any specified period of time or to make any agreement contrary to the foregoing.

I further understand that any offer of employment tendered as a result of this application is contingent upon successful completion of the following: a pre-employment post-offer drug screen, a fitness-for-duty assessment, verification of legal right to work in the United States, previous employment history, history of arrest and conviction, verification of education, professional licenses and certifications, personal references, and motor vehicle records.

By signing this application, I authorize [Practice Name] and its agents to investigate information I have given in this application, resume, or during the interview process and to conduct a background investigation. I hereby release all claims against [Practice Name] and its respective employees, officers, trustees, agents, and any person or agent supplying information that might arise out of the aforementioned investigation. I have received a "Disclosure Statement— Notice to Applicant of Intent to Obtain a Consumer Report." I have signed a "Release to Procure a Consumer Report."

This application when completed and signed becomes the property of [*Practice Name*].

_____   _____
Applicant's Signature   Date

_____
Applicant's Name (Please Print)

Performing Reference and Background Checks

It is imperative that reference and/or background checks be conducted for each new employee you are considering hiring. At least three references should be checked by requesting either a letter or telephone interview that discusses the applicant's job history and skills. The primary reason for conducting checks is to ensure that the applicant's data are reliable and also to obtain the perceptions of previous employees or teachers regarding the employee's own record.

Bernardin and Russell also note that fear of negligent hiring is a related reason employers conduct checks of reference and background. In *Human Resource Management: An Experiential Approach*, Bernardin and Russell cite an example of an HMO that was sued for $10 million when a patient under the care of a psychologist was committed to a hospital and it was later revealed that the psychologist not only was unlicensed but also lied about his previous experience.[6] Attempting to accelerate the hiring process by forgoing prudent screening could cost more in the long run.

Another reason to check references is to attempt to ascertain if the potential hire will be able to succeed and grow into the job and contribute to the work environment in a positive manner. Physicians must recognize that each member of their practice plays an integral role in the profitability and success of the practice.

Bernardin and Russell also state that background checks should include police records, particularly convictions, and driving records, if applicable. If physicians are uncomfortable with letters of reference, which tend to be mostly positive, Bernardin and Russell advocate constructing a "letter of reference," or a recommendation that is essentially a performance appraisal form. They also suggest constructing a rating form and requesting that the evaluator indicate the extent to which the candidate was effective in performing a list of job tasks.

Although it appears to be cumbersome, physicians and/or medical office managers should attempt to do their best in obtaining valid reference checks. As Bernardin and Russell note, a good-faith effort to obtain verification of employment history can make it possible for a company to avoid (or win) negligent hiring lawsuits.

Conducting Interviews

The employment interview is still the most utilized tool for selecting employees. Following is a list of suggestions offered by Bernardin and Russell to help physicians and/or office managers conduct meaningful, effective employment interviews:

1. Exclude traits that can be measured by more valid employment tests, such as intelligence, job attitudes or ability, job skills, or knowledge.

2. Include motivational and interpersonal factors that are required for effective job performance. These two areas seem to have the most potential for both overall and interviewer validity. Interviewers should assess only those factors that are specifically exhibited in the behavior of the applicant during the interview and are critical for performance in the job to be filled.

3. Match interview questions (content areas) with the job analysis data of the job to be filled and the strategic goals of the organization.

4. Avoid biased language and jokes that may detract from the formality of the interview, and inquiries that are not relevant to the job in question.

5. Limit the amount of preinterview information to complete about the applicants' qualifications and clear up any ambiguous data. While knowledge of test results, letters of reference, and other sources of information can bias an interview, it is a good strategy to seek additional information relevant to applicants' levels of KASOCs. (See "Establishing Job Descriptions" earlier in this chapter for a definition of *KASOC*.)

Sample Disclosure Statement and Release Form

Notice to Applicant of Intent to Obtain a Consumer Report

By this document, [*Practice Name*] discloses the following to you. A consumer report may be obtained for employment purposes as part of the pre-employment background investigation and at any time during your employment.

> *A consumer report may include driving records, criminal arrests and convictions, prior employment history, verification of education, professional licenses and certifications, and other public record information.*

Before we may procure a consumer report, you must authorize such procurement in writing. You have the right to decline authorization for us to procure a consumer report. However, we will not consider you further for employment if you so decline.

On an attached form, you will find a release that will allow [*Practice* Name] to obtain a consumer report. Please read the release carefully before signing it and indicating your choice regarding disclosure.

Release to Procure a Consumer Report

I have read the "Notice to Applicant of Intent to Obtain Consumer Report" letter. I understand that I have the right to decline authorization for [*Practice Name*] to procure a consumer report concerning me.

I understand that the consumer report may contain information concerning criminal arrests and convictions, driving records, prior employment history, verification of education, and professional licenses and certifications.

I understand that, if hired, this authorization shall remain on file and shall serve as an ongoing authorization to procure consumer reports at any time during my employment period. Therefore, understanding these rights,

I (circle one) <u>AUTHORIZE / DO NOT AUTHORIZE</u> [*Practice Name*] to procure a consumer report concerning me.

_____

Applicant Name (Please Print)

_____   _____

Signature   Date

_____

Human Resources Representative

Many interviews are unstructured. These are usually characterized by open-ended questions that are not based on or associated with the job. However, research illustrates that structured interviews can improve the reliability and validity of the process.

Elaine Pulakos and Neal Schmitt studied experience-based and situational interviews in "Experience-Based and Situational Interview Questions: Studies of Validity."[7] They define experience-based interviews in which questions are *post-oriented* in that they ask the respondents to relate what they did in past jobs or life situations that is relevant to a particular job—relevant knowledge, skills, and abilities of successful employees. For example, "Think about a time when you had to motivate an employee to perform a job task that he or she disliked but that you needed the individual to do. How did you handle the situation?"

A situational interview question asks the job applicant to imagine a set of circumstances and then indicate how he or she would respond in that situation; hence, the questions are *future-oriented*. For example, "Suppose you were working with an employee who you knew greatly disliked performing a particular job task. You were in a situation where you needed this task completed, and this employee was the only person available to assist you. What would you do to motivate the employee to perform the task?"

Pulakos and Schmitt found that the experience-based interviews were more valid than the situational interviews under their tightly controlled experimental conditions. However, research suggests that using structured interviews rather than unstructured interviews obtains results with better reliability and validity.

Employees must also have the skills for the job and they must be encouraged to continue their education on the job. Bernardin and Russell acknowledge that companies are interested in selecting employees not only who will be effective, but who will also work as long as the companies want them, and who will not engage in counterproductive behavior, such as violence, substance abuse, avoidable accidents, and employee theft.

Personnel may account for a major portion of the physician office budget, but it is the personnel that are essential for the long-run success of any physician practice. Therefore, while it might seem cumbersome, it is crucial that time and money are allocated to recruit and retain the best employees.

Today's work environment has numerous employers competing for employees who can help make or break a practice.

Endnotes

1. Bernardin J, Russell J. *Human Resource Management: An Experiential Approach, Second Edition.* Boston, MA: Irwin/McGraw-Hill; 1998.

2. Moos R. *Work Environmental Scale Manual.* Palo Alto, CA: Consulting Psychologists Press; 1994.

3. Rokeach M. *Rokeach Value Survey.* Palo Alto, CA: Consulting Psychologists Press; 1988.

4. Jay D. *The Essential Personnel Sourcebook, Second Edition.* London, UK: Financial Times Management; 1998.

5. Lawson WR. *How to Develop a Personnel Policy Manual.* New York: AMACOM; 1998.

6. Bernardin J, Russell J. *Human Resource Management: An Experiential Approach, Second Edition.* Boston, MA: Irwin/McGraw-Hill; 1998.

7. Pulakos E, Schmitt N. Experience-based and situational interview questions: studies of validity, *Personnel Psychology*; 1995.

Chapter 4

Should You Purchase or Lease?

*D*r Brown resigned his position as a staff radiologist at Anywhere General Hospital and elected to open his own diagnostic imaging center. He met with his accountant and left the meeting more confused than he was when he went in. The accountant asked him a number of questions regarding financing the startup. Dr Brown had assumed he would use his personal savings as a downpayment and finance the balance. However, the accountant explained to Dr Brown that he could lease staff, real estate, and equipment, or he could hire employees directly and purchase the office building and the equipment. He explained the pros and cons of each scenario and asked Dr Brown to make a decision. Dr Brown left the accountant's office unsure of what decision to make.

Cost containment is a critical issue in medical practices facing declining revenue and increased operational costs. The decision to lease or purchase the practice facilities has a tremendous impact on the future overhead of any medical practice.

Starting a new practice, expanding an existing practice, or just replacing worn equipment and furnishing requires much greater analysis than would be expected. In the past, physicians wanting to accomplish any of the previously mentioned tasks could pick up the telephone, call his or her banker, and arrange a loan. That approach once worked, but in today's tumultuous health care environment a physician might be shocked at the response of the lending institution.

Many lenders are no longer the local banks with which the physician had a friendly relationship. Today, the physician often faces large conglomerates that follow strict rules and no longer employ "Mom and Pop" relationships as part of their banking strategies. As a matter of fact, new physicians entering practice for the first time may be surprised at the difficulty they face in borrowing money for their startup.

In addition to the complexities of borrowing money, physicians face perplexing issues related to hiring and managing staff for the practice. Most physicians are not trained in human resource management, may not know how to properly conduct interviews, and are usually unaware of the myriad state and federal regulations that must be followed in managing a staff of employees.

A fairly recent option that is available to physicians is *leasing* employees. This option and its consequences are discussed in this chapter. Remember: the decision to lease or purchase has significant long-range consequences that cannot be easily reversed. These consequences include federal and state tax implications that must be reviewed with the practice accountant.

Figure 4.1 provides a summary of the factors involved in making the "lease versus buy" decision, highlighting the key factors that play a role in this complex process.

Figure 4.1: A Summary of Factors Involved in Making the Lease versus Buy Decision

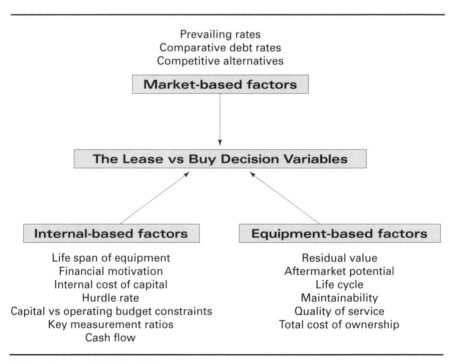

Prevailing rates
Comparative debt rates
Competitive alternatives

Market-based factors

The Lease vs Buy Decision Variables

Internal-based factors

Life span of equipment
Financial motivation
Internal cost of capital
Hurdle rate
Capital vs operating budget constraints
Key measurement ratios
Cash flow

Equipment-based factors

Residual value
Aftermarket potential
Life cycle
Maintainability
Quality of service
Total cost of ownership

Selecting What You Want

The first step in deciding whether to lease or purchase the necessary equipment to run your practice is to decide what item the practice wishes to obtain and the specific brand that is desired. In order to accomplish this critical step, you must determine what features you want and exactly what you want the equipment to do.

The best place to start is to develop a *request for information* (RFI) and/or a *request for proposal* (RFP). This document can then be sent to three to five vendors. Once the vendors' responses are received, the practice should develop a spreadsheet so that all of the vendors can be compared feature by feature. When you have entered all of the responses to your RFI/RFP, you will easily be able to eliminate the vendors that don't meet your criteria.

The next step is to compare prices for each of the vendors that meet all of your preestablished criteria. You should then request a list of references from comparable practices that you can contact. Always contact the reference without the sales representative present. If the company representative insists on participating in the reference review, assume that they have something to hide and eliminate that vendor from your list of finalists.

Now, you are almost ready to make your selection. The last step is to review the financing aspect of your purchase. Most vendors will have leasing options available. Of course, you always have the option of making an outright purchase. This decision is the focus of our discussion.

When reviewing your options for the choice of equipment and the best price, make sure you also explore the purchasing cooperatives available to you. In many instances, local medical

This chapter focuses on cost containment and the factors that influence the financial viability of a medical practice. None of the authors is qualified to practice accountancy. Therefore, the purpose of mentioning these issues is to create awareness of issues that will have a significant impact on the viability of a medical practice. Prior to making decisions that have long-range financial implications, we strongly suggest you seek the advice of a qualified professional.

societies, medical specialty societies, independent practice associations (IPAs), hospital associations, chambers of commerce, and other groups have established purchasing alliances. Some of these purchasing alliances have arrangements with certain vendors for discounts on their products. These arrangements will take a lot of the hard work and research out of the purchasing process.

It is important to review warranties that are provided for the various items you are reviewing. Most of the warranties are similar, but they will not be identical. The terms of the warranties may be a key decision-maker.

Leasing Equipment

A good way to begin a discussion of leasing equipment is to review basic terminology. Leasing can be a confusing process that is filled with a language of its own.

Who's Who

The *lessor* is the party who owns the asset. The *lessee* is the party who rents the asset.

Types of Leases

There are two types of leases a physician may encounter: a capital lease and an operating lease.

- A *capital lease* is one in which the physician is planning a long-term commitment to utilize the asset, possibly for the life of the asset. This type of lease brings with it legal and accounting questions.

- An *operating lease* is utilized when an asset is needed on a short-term basis or the asset involves rapidly advancing technology that will render it obsolete in a relatively short time. The real question with an operating lease is how well you can negotiate advantageous terms.

Depreciation

Based on the advice of your accountant, leasing can be an excellent strategy for a medical practice. The key considerations involved in leasing are the availability of capital to make a purchase, the personal tax implications for the physician and for the practice as a business entity, and the long-range strategy that is being fulfilled. However, in addition to these issues, the physician must also consider depreciation.

Depreciation is the accounting and tax recognition of the decline in the value of an asset. It is an accounting number, not a cash flow. Depreciation expense offers a tax benefit to those who own assets; thus, a key factor in the decision to lease equipment is to weigh the tax benefit of utilizing depreciation versus writing off the lease payments.[1]

Conducting Due Diligence

In "Nine Things the Equipment-Leasing Salesman Won't Tell You," Milton Zall discusses some of the lesser-known facts of leasing[2]:

- Leasing isn't necessarily cheaper than buying.

- Any tax advantage will be outweighed by higher leasing costs.

- Leasing doesn't tie up your capital or credit line.

- You could be personally liable for fulfilling the lease.

- Leasing does not make your balance sheet look better.

- Leasing represents a commitment you may come to regret.

- The company may not like the condition of the equipment when your lease ends.

- The contract could contain a tax trap.

- The leasing company won't remind you when your lease expires.

Do these points mean that you should not lease because all leases are bad? No. Rather, the author points out that the leasing company is not looking out for the lessees' interests. Therefore, prior to entering into a lease, you should conduct a thorough due diligence process. This process begins by utilizing professionals, such as your accountant, to assist in determining the financial implications of leasing versus purchasing. In addition, legal counsel should review all lease documents prior to final execution of the document.

Financing

It cannot be emphasized enough that the financing option should match the use of the equipment being financed. If careful consideration is not given to all aspects of these choices, the practice may make some very costly mistakes. In "Analyzing Lease Purchase Options," an article that appeared in *Radiology Management*, David Cioleck and James Mace offer the following rules to guide the lease versus buy process[3]:

- Use the *purchase* alternative for assets that are certain to remain in the organization past their projected residual value life, without increasing the total cost of operation costs of retaining the asset to an unacceptable level.

- When the sole purpose is to preserve cash, but the same certainty of life within the organization exists as with the purchase alternative above, choose *finance* or *sales-type leases* (eg, $1 buyout, fixed balloon buyout, other fixed financing structures). Choose a lease term that is as well matched to the projected useful life as possible.

- If an identifiable term of use for the equipment is less than its full projected useful life, but preserving cash flow, limiting capital budgets, and keeping nonearning assets off the books are motivators, select a *fair market value lease* with an operating lease structure. However, choose a lease term to match how long it is projected to remain at your organization without major regard for the marketable life of the equipment.

- If uncertainty exists around the term of use within the organization or in the underlying technology of the equipment (rapidly changing technology), choose a *fair market value lease with a buyout range* (eg, a floor and a cap) or agreed upon renewal terms.

Office Space: Buy or Rent?

Many physicians in a private practice have a strong desire to own their office space. They believe that because they spend most of their working hours in the office, it would be better to own the space and not pay rent month after month. In most instances this is an emotional reaction that is not based on a financial analysis of this option.

Owning a medical office building may sound like an excellent strategy, but small commercial office buildings are not, in most cases, a good investment, as these properties can be difficult to rent or sell. The same funds invested in other financial instruments can yield a much higher return.

One of the key problems with a physician owning his or her own office building is that the physician is locked into an existing facility. The physician cannot make the building bigger if the practice grows and requires more space or, conversely, the physician cannot decide to use a much smaller space if he or she downsizes the practice. Linked to these issues is the fact that, over time, geographic areas change and the physician may want to move the practice or, even worse, the tenants decide to relocate because of population shifts or other related factors.

In today's environment many doctors use multiple sites for their practice. This means that a physician may only practice at a given location once or twice a week. It makes more sense to establish relationships with other physicians who can sublet the space, thereby reducing overhead, than to acquire the building and be locked into a situation that does not meet the needs of the practice.

Property management and ownership is a time-consuming and costly activity, and most physicians are too busy with their existing work schedules and personal lives to properly attend to it. Adding the significant responsibility of being a landlord will keep physicians from their patients and primary source of revenue, put physicians in a business where they most likely have no training or experience, and expose them to financial risk. If a physician is considering purchasing his or her office space, he or she should review this option carefully with professional advisors to weigh the personal and financial risks involved.

Leasing Staff

Cost containment can be accomplished in various ways. One of the methodologies gaining significant attention is *outsourcing*. Outsourcing of various practice functions can help contain costs, even though it may not initially bring with it a reduction in cost. By outsourcing, the physician can focus on the primary business of patient care and allow others to deal with the complex management issues that abound in the practice. Outsourcing of various medical practice functions is not a new concept in the health care industry—hospitals have outsourced numerous functions, such as house-keeping, for many years.

The outsourcing function of interest in this discussion is *employee leasing.* Employee leasing has become a booming industry that targets small businesses, making physician practices a prime target. There are advantages and disadvantages to outsourcing your practice employees, and you should investigate this thoroughly before considering a major shift in the management of your practice.

Employee leasing is accomplished by retaining a firm that will "lease" the employees of the practice that hired them. The leasing firm, for a fee of about 2% to 8% of total payroll costs, assumes the human resource management and all associated personnel paperwork. The employee leasing firm will assume responsibility for payroll administration, benefit administration, unemployment compensation, and compliance with federal and state labor laws.

From the perspective of busy physicians, leasing staff makes it possible to reduce workload in an area that is almost always rife with problems. For all practical purposes, the physician retains management control of the staff and the employee leasing company retains control of the human resource functions. The doctor writes one check per month to the employee leasing firm and that organization assumes responsibilities for all payroll and employee benefit payments.

Jay Finegan, author of the *Inc.* magazine article "Look Before You Lease," offers some criteria for consideration when considering employee leasing[4]:

- Complete a due diligence process on the employee leasing company and be sure they are financially solvent.

- Request a long list of references and contact each one personally.

- Make sure you are comfortable with the employee leasing company.

- Be sure of the services that are available and that they meet your needs.

- Have the contract reviewed by legal counsel to ensure that the practice is amply protected.

The decision to lease employees is complex. First, the physician must be sure that this type of arrangement will blend with his or her management style and needs. Second, the physician must be sure that employee leasing makes financial sense for the practice. Third, outsourcing of services is not for everyone. Some physicians are content with only managing the clinical aspect of the practice, while others become extremely frustrated with dealing with an additional tier of management to accomplish tasks that were completely under their control in the past.

If employee leasing is a consideration, it is important to shop around for the best deal: one that accomplishes all of the practice goals and objectives, not necessarily the one that is the cheapest. Negotiate and get what you want or do not undertake employee leasing.

Negotiating Leases

Negotiating is a critical skill in the management of any business. In a medical practice that is diligently working toward financial success, negotiating becomes critical. From a cost containment perspective, a poorly negotiated lease can have a disastrous impact on the practice bottom line for years after the lease is signed. It is imperative that physicians culminate their search and negotiation with the best lease terms available.

Prior to starting the search for new equipment, or whatever is being leased, the physician should complete a due diligence process. This process should include the following:

- An understanding of what additional debt service the practice can manage on a monthly basis.

- A definition of what the practice specifically is trying to accomplish and why.

- A definition of the terms the practice willing to accept (such as 3, 5, or 10-year amortization of the note, small payments with a balloon payment at the end of the lease, a number of months with no payment, and so on).

- Assurances that the lease terms take seasonal fluctuations in patient volume and cash flow into consideration. Understand the life of the proposed equipment and make sure a lessor allows for upgrades of the equipment during the life of the lease.

- A review your own credit and the practice's credit. Make sure you know where you stand, because the strength of your credit will determine how good a deal is obtained and the strength of your negotiating position.

Compare Lessors

Once the basics have been mapped out, the practice is ready to begin shopping for leases. It is critical that a number of lessors be contacted and compared for the best rates and terms. Do not rely on the equipment vendor or manufacturer to provide the optimal leasing package.

The simplest way to compare lessors is to create a spreadsheet and compare the features of each financing option offered. This is a simple way of matching the features and terms of each lease by scanning your spreadsheet. This spreadsheet could be very simply taken to the next step and turned into an RFI or an RFP. The data obtained from these requests could then be plugged into the spreadsheet for comparative purposes.

It is important to remember that each financial organization will have variations in its leases. During your review of leases it is important to watch for hidden costs that have been placed in the lease.

Upon completion of your lease review, there is one more important step: *Do not accept the service agreement that is offered with an equipment lease*, as it will not always be the most comprehensive or cost-effective. Shop around for third-party vendor service agreements. The practice may be able to obtain a service contract for up to 35% to 60% less than those offered by the original equipment manufacturer.

During the due diligence process, there is nothing wrong in letting lessors know they are competing for your business. Never be afraid to ask for the terms you would like in the lease. In many instances, the lessor may be flexible in order to make a sale.

Review Documents

Finally, at the end of the negotiating process, the selected lessor will provide you with multiple documents for signature. It is extremely important that every document be carefully reviewed and fully understood prior to signing. It is also strongly recommended that the practice have legal counsel review these documents and offer suggested enhancements or changes. Often the attorneys' suggestions can be incorporated into the lease. There may also be times when a contract is so onerous that the wise decision is to say no and select a different lessor. Remember, if it sounds too good to be true, it probably is!

Purchasing

The decision to purchase equipment is somewhat simpler to carry out than the decision to lease. If you have decided to buy then you have eliminated the concerns associated with the complexities of leasing. But an astute buyer will look at numerous issues that apply to the buying cycle.

After deciding to buy a specific item, whether small or a capital purchase, the potential buyer must look at several critical issues, including the following:

- Should the purchase be for cash taken from operations or the physicians' personal savings?

- Should the purchase be financed through a loan to the practice?

- What about service contracts?

- Where do I go for the best deal?

Purchasing is a complex process that follows a similar format to leasing. In reality, the process that is followed should be identical to leasing, up to the point of paying for the purchase. As discussed earlier, you should go through a due diligence process and make a determination as to the best source of funds for you to utilize in making your purchase.

Decision Factors

There are several key factors that may slant the decision process to a buying scenario. The first of these factors, and probably the most important, is the impact on cash flow. It is important to review the lease or buy options and determine which will have the least negative impact on cash flow for the practice. This is accomplished by preparing a lease versus buy analysis chart. The bottom line of this analysis will reveal the best option.

Another critical issue in purchasing is to determine the potential value of the equipment after 5 years of use. If the equipment is worth more than 10% of the original purchase price, buying may be a viable option. Generally, a good rule of thumb is to not buy high-tech equipment or equipment that is evolving very rapidly. For example, it makes more sense to purchase x-ray equipment, which rarely makes major changes, than to purchase magnetic resonance imaging (MRI) equipment, where the technology is rapidly advancing and obsolescence is a constant reality.

The next issue for review is depreciation. In almost all instances, lessees are unable to depreciate the equipment they have leased. However, a buyer can fully depreciate the equipment over a period of time and expense the amount depreciated each year. It is important to have your accountant review this aspect of a purchase before you make a final decision.

Finally, when purchasing, the buyer must review the sales tax consequence and compare it to the taxes that are placed on a lease. Sales tax issues will vary from state to state; thus, it is important to have your accountant analyze the consequences of either decision.

The most widely used comparison is the lease versus purchase internal rate of return (IRR) produced by measuring the cash flow of the purchase case compared to the cash flow of the lease case.[5] The number that results is a measure of the rate of return of using your money for one scenario or the other. As the number gets higher, the concept of purchasing becomes more attractive. Figure 4.2 illustrates an example of a methodology that can be used for comparing two options that are available.

Figure 4.2: The After-Tax Purchase Comparison versus Leasing

Example Model: 3-Year Term
Leasing Costs
Initial purchase price $1,000

Purhase vs lease comparison	Rate	Initial Cost	Year 1	Year 2	Year 3	Total
Lease cost						
Base monthly lease cost w/use tax	6%	$1,000.00				
Annual leasing cost	0.02895		$368.24	$368.24	$368.24	$1,104.73
Taxes	38%		($139.93)	($139.93)	($139.93)	$419.80
Net annual leasing cost			$228.31	$228.31	$228.31	$684.93
Purchase cost						
Cost		$1,000.00	$0.00	$0.00	$0.00	$1,000.00
Book expenses						
Sales tax-capital	6.00%	$60.00				
Depreciation	3		$212.00	$339.20	$203.52	$754.72
Book (gain)/loss of sale			$0.00	$0.00	$235.16	$235.16
Taxes			($80.56)	($128.90)	($166.70)	($376.15)
After-tax purchase cost of funds	7.00%		$74.20	$59.36	$35.62	$169.18
Total initial cost		$1,060.00				
Net annual book expense			$205.64	$269.66	$307.59	$782.90
Net income impact						
Leasing cost			$228.31	$228.31	$228.31	$684.93
Purchase cost			$205.64	$269.66	$307.59	$782.90
Purchase vs lease book expense benefit			$22.67	($41.35)	$79.28	($97.96)
Cash flow impact						
Of leasing—annual leasing cost			($228.31)	($228.31)	($228.31)	($684.93)
Net cash flow of leasing		$0 00	($228.31)	($228.31)	($228.31)	($684.93)
Of purchasing						
Book expense			($205.64)	($269.66)	($307.59)	($782.90)
Add non-cash expenses—depreciation			$212.00	$339.20	$203.52	$754.72
Add non-cash expenses—gain/loss			$0.00	$0.00	$235.16	$235.16
Subtract non-book items—total initial cost		($1,060.00)	$0.00	$0.00	$0.00	($1,060.00)
Add sale of equipment proceeds			$0.00	$0.00	$70.13	$70.13
Subtract taxes on gain on sale					$0.00	$0.00
Net cash flow of purchase		($1,060.00)	$6.36	$69.54	$201.21	($614.81)
Cash flow impact of purchase vs lease		($1,060.00)	$234.67	$297.85	$429.52	($97.96)
Purchase payback		$1,060.00	$825.33	$527.48	$97.96	
Payback period (years)	3.2		1.0	1.0	1.2	
Net present value of purchase		0	1	2	3	
vs lease cash flow	−5.4%	($1,060.00)	$241.00	$324.00	$494.00	$0.00
Purchase vs lease IRR	−5.47%					

Endnotes

1. Bukics RM, Chambers, DR. *Medical Practice Accounting & Finance: A Practical Guide for Physicians, Dentists, and Other Medical Practitioners.* New York, NY: Probus Publishing; 1995.

2. Zall M. Nine things the equipment-leasing salesman won't tell you. *Physician's Management.* April 1998.

3. Cioleck D, Mace J. Equipment acquisition using various forms of leasing. *Radiology Management.* May/June 1998.

4. Finegan J. Look before you lease. *Inc.* February 1997.

5. Cioleck D, Mace J. Analyzing lease purchase options. *Radiology Management.* May/June 1998.

Chapter 5

Selecting and Working With Consultants

Good consultants can help increase productivity, provide innovative ideas and services, and cut or contain costs. They can help reduce paperwork, ensure compliance with various regulations, and help with staffing issues and concerns.

Hiring a Consultant

Following are six suggestions for working with consultants:

1. **Be proactive.** Line up help before you need it. Search out various consultants you need immediately and those you may need later.

2. **Start from the middle and work toward the top.** The difference between the "middle" and the "top" consultants may not be worth their differences in cost. Often, qualified, knowledgeable consultants looking to grow might be more cost-effective and practice attentive. That is, major problems and issues within the practice, if identified early, may not need high-priced, big-name consulting firms. (And often the work at the big names is handled by less senior personnel anyway.) Therefore, why pay for the embellishments of these high-priced consultants when others will do?

3. **Check and recheck references.** Be sure to ask for and check references. It is also important to check various regulating bodies and peer review groups when available to ensure the reliability and track record of any consultant.

4. **Communicate constantly with the consultant(s).** Let consultants know how the practice is progressing. Any major changes should be shared with the consultants.

5. **Always review and re-review the consultant's advice.** In most cases, advice should be followed, but if physicians find the advice unhelpful or detrimental they should not be afraid to speak with the consultant and, if needed, look for a replacement.

6. **Consultants work for the physician; not vice versa.** Be demanding and make clear what you expect. You are paying for the services of the consultant, so you should be satisfied with his or her work. The worst situation is to be unhappy or disappointed with a consultant and to not maximize efficiency and profitability.

In "Don't Ask the Questions if You Don't Want to Know the Answer," an article that appeared in *Physician Executive*, Daniel Zabel and Ronald Kaufman note that outside expertise is sought for one or more of the following reasons:

- The lack of "in-house" personnel or time to deliver a product.

- The need for an external expert to bring credibility to the project.

- Getting someone outside your organization to deliver unpopular or bad news.

- A genuine interest in the independent findings and recommendations of the consultant.

Zabel and Kaufman further note that "whatever the motivation for seeking the advice of outside counsel, be sure you are prepared for the answer they may give to the question you asked."[1]

Some of the experts physicians may need to consider consulting include bankers, accountants, attorneys, and health care consultants.

Consultants Checklist

Following is a checklist to use when selecting various consultants for your practice. It can provide a means to compare different consultants and help narrow the choices.

Chemistry: _____

_____

Education: _____

_____

Experience: _____

_____

Training: _____

_____

Philosophy: _____

_____

Resources: _____

_____

Areas of Interest: _____

_____

Professional and Community Involvement: _____

_____

Type and Size of Firm: _____

_____

Schedule: _____

_____

References: _____

_____

Honors/Awards: _____

_____

Value Survey: _____

_____

Experience-Based Situations: _____

_____

Bankers

Physicians and medical office managers should have at least one local banker, and they should consider retaining one or two national bankers. Often, bankers are one of the first professionals physicians consult because they can help in financing the physician practice. Bankers can establish lines of credit and can be a great vehicle for obtaining local business information and providing contacts.

Accountants

Before selecting a certified public accountant (CPA) for your practice, it is important to do your research. The National CPA Health Care Advisors Association (www.hcaa.com) recommends researching the following criteria before selecting a CPA: expertise, education, training, resources, area(s) of concentration, professional and community involvement, size of the firm, price, chemistry, and references. For example, following are a few of the questions a physician should ask a CPA before making the decision to hire him or her:

- How many years' experience does the CPA have and with what type of health care clients?

- What degrees did the CPA earn?

- How much continuing professional education (CPE) did the accountant earn? When and where?

- Where did the CPE earn his or her credits in the past 5 years? How much work was in health care?

- Who does the CPA use for researching potential problems?

Physicians most often need CPAs who do a significant amount of work in health care. And, with all of the changes occurring in health care, physicians should know what CPAs do to stay abreast of changes. It is also important to know what, if any, professional and trade organizations the CPA belongs to. For example, is he or she a member of the National CPA Health Care Advisors Association, the Medical Group Management Association, American College of Health Care Executives, or the American College of Health Care Administrators? Physicians should also know what type of involvement and participation the CPA has in such professional organizations and the community. For example, does the CPA hold any leadership roles?

In addition, physicians must decide if they want to work with a sole practitioner or a CPA associated with a small, medium, or large firm. Physicians should also consider whether they need a regional, national, or international firm.

Physicians also must have the CPA explain the billing fees and procedures, which should be held in writing and provide answers to such questions as, when support staff is used will this be billed at a different rate? What are these rates?

One of the most important criteria in selecting and retaining CPAs is the chemistry between the CPA and the physician and the medical office manager. In addition to many of the criteria mentioned above, none of it will matter if the physician and CPA do not have a good working relationship. Poor chemistry can only result in an inefficient and costly relationship.

Physicians should review at least three CPAs before making their final selection, and those CPAs should have letters of reference from health care clients.[2] A good place to find potential CPAs is from referrals from friends, bankers, or other consultants, or seeking names from national groups such as the National CPA Health Care Advisors Association.

Attorneys

There are plenty of attorneys to choose from; however, physicians should be prudent about whom they select. Proper selection of attorneys has saved physicians and their practices thousands of dollars.

In *The Upstart Small Business Legal Guide, Second Edition*,[3] Robert Friedman suggests asking attorneys the following questions:

- What is your experience with the type of legal matter that I have?

- What are your initial consultation fee and hourly rates?

- Have you lectured at services held for the general public or other attorneys or written books or articles?

- How many attorneys are in your firm? Is it a full-service firm?

- What days and hours is the office open?

- Does the firm have specialists? If so, in what areas? (While in some states attorneys cannot hold themselves out as specialists, they may still state that their practice is "limited" to a certain area of the law, such as divorce, corporate, or criminal.)

- What percentage of your practice is devoted to my type of legal problem?

- Does the firm provide tax preparation and tax planning?

- Does the firm publish a client newsletter in which it explains new developments in the law? Are informational pamphlets on the law available?

- Is the attorney familiar with the following areas of federal and state law: income and estate taxation, corporation, aging, partnership, securities, antitrust, contracts, and product liability?

- Does the attorney have knowledge and experience with such nonlegal concepts as corporate finance, financial accounting, management technologies, and how to work with bankers, brokers, insurers, and industrial development agencies?

Friedman also discusses the importance of preventive legal audits (PLA). PLAs are comprehensive appraisals of a physician practice's legal affairs whereby attorneys can make constructive recommendations for changes in physician practice policies and procedures. Friedman states that annual PLAs can help clients do the following:

- Avoid jail and fines

- Avoid court

- Reduce legal costs

- Improve their reputation and public relations

- Take advantage of future trends

- Educate their employees

- Improve their work environment

According to Friedman, attorneys who conduct PLAs should visit a practice, analyze the practice's legal vulnerability, and draft a remedial plan for the client explaining potential legal exposure.[3]

Health Care Consultants

Physicians may also elicit the help of health care consultants to assess the practice's work environment and recommend ways for increasing the practice's organizational efficiency and effectiveness. Some of the best places for selecting consultants include:

- American Association of Healthcare Consultants (www.aahc.net)

- Medical Group Management Association (www.mgma.com)

- The Society for Healthcare Strategy and Market Development (www.stratsociety.org)

Physicians should follow the same steps that are used in selecting bankers, accountants, and attorneys, making sure to ask health care consultants for specific successful cases and turnaround situations.

Endnotes

1. Zabel D, Kaufman R. Don't ask the questions if you don't want to know the answer, *Physician Executive*. 1995.

2. American Association of Healthcare Consultants (www.aahc.net).

3. Friedman R. *The Upstart Small Business Legal Guide, Second Edition*. Chicago, IL: Dearborn Financial Publishing; 1998.

Chapter 6

Recruiting and Retaining Practitioners

The decision to add an additional practitioner to a practice can be a difficult one, and one that comes with significant cost considerations. Before making such a decision there are numerous issues to examine. And, once you have made the decision to add a practitioner, whether a physician extender or a full- or part-time physician, how you go about the process will also affect your costs. This chapter looks at the decision-making process and explores cost considerations inherent in the decision to increase staff.

Determining a Need for Additional Staff

There are many reasons for adding help to a practice. The most obvious is to handle a rising demand for medical services experienced by the practice. When patients must wait weeks or even months for an appointment, or when the practice will no longer accept new patients because of the demand of current patients, there is clear indication that the current system is overloaded, being run inefficiently, or not meeting the needs of the community. Both situations can signal the need to consider adding an additional practitioner. But there are other reasons to consider this step.

Help With Patient Volume

In some practices, senior physicians may wish to slow down and work limited schedules. Other physicians may wish to pursue opportunities both in and out of medicine that will require additional help with the patient volume. These, too, will require the addition of practitioners.

Creation of a Multispecialty Practice

At some point, the volume of referrals a practice makes to other physicians in a specific specialty may become great enough to warrant the addition of that physician or other provider to perform those services within the practice. It is not unusual for a busy practice to refer a significant number of patients for specific treatments or procedures not currently provided in the practice. In reviewing the referrals a practice makes to other physicians, an opportunity to retain those patients and the attendant revenue may exist, thereby expanding the scope of the services offered by the practice. This can be the beginning of a multispecialty practice.

Deciding to Add Staff

The decision to add staff to a practice should not be made lightly. The current practice operations should be carefully analyzed to determine whether such a move makes financial and practical sense. In addition, efficiency of operations should be evaluated. In many cases, changes in the practice's patient flow and scheduling may solve the demand for care. Analysis of unmet needs can also indicate alternatives to adding new staff. Don't jump to conclusions based on anecdotal information.

If, after careful review, it is apparent that the practice should consider adding a practitioner or other staff, the rest of this chapter can help determine the course of action and identify cost containment considerations for the process.

Adding Physician Extenders

The use of physician extenders—such as physician assistants and nurse practitioners—has increased in recent years for many reasons. Pressure from managed care organizations to increase access coupled with reduced reimbursement has been one factor. The need to provide care in medically underserved areas is another. The use of physician extenders in a practice also helps to maintain the necessary volume of all patients in a practice: with physician extenders, physicians are able to see patients with more serious medical conditions while physician extenders handle more of the routine care.

The decision to use a physician extender must be made carefully and only after a detailed analysis of the practice's needs and the role and limitation of the extender. If an extender can provide the care needed, the practice can see significant cost savings. In addition, the cost to recruit physician extenders is generally lower than that of a physician.

Types of Physician Extenders

There are several types of physician extenders working in physician practices throughout the United States. Some are trained in specific fields, such as optometrists (who may work in an ophthalmologist office to provide refractive services) or chiropractors (who may be hired by orthopedic surgeons to provide manipulation services). Others provide a broader range of patient services. It is this category of physician extenders that is seeing a great growth in demand. The two principal types of extenders in this category are physician assistants (PAs) and nurse practitioners (NPs).

PAs and NPs can provide a cost-effective means of expanding a practice's volume. However, care must be used to determine whether these extenders are able to provide the care needed to meet the demand for growth in the practice. To make this determination, you must look at the limitations of PAs and NPs and carefully analyze the services your practice is providing.

Limitation of Extenders

The care physician extenders can give is limited by several entities. The limitations may be created by state statutes, which regulate the practice of the extenders, and by third-party payors, who may specify limitations on reimbursement.

Before considering the use of physician extenders, carefully review the limitations. Start with the state law and regulations that identify the specific and general areas in which an extender can be used. Determine whether the laws in your state allow the use of physician extenders in the areas in which you wish to use them.

You may review the state laws yourself or contact the professional society for the particular

Separate laws govern PAs and NPs, and these laws vary between states. For example, only the state of Mississippi disallows the use of PAs in all practices except in federal facilities.

physician extender. These societies will be glad to inform you of the services that the extender can provide and under what circumstances.

It is also important to check with the various third-party payors for which you provide care to ascertain what services are covered and what the reimbursement will be. Some third-party payors may also impose additional limits on the use of extenders. Make sure you get this information in writing and seek any necessary clarification.

General Uses of Extenders

Physician extenders, including PAs and NPs, can practice in a variety of settings. Again, their roles may be limited by state law or by third-party payors, but generally, they work effectively in most outpatient settings including offices, clinics, nursing homes, and so on. They can perform physical examinations, order laboratory tests, diagnose and treat illnesses, suture wounds, and assist in surgery. Many states allow PAs and NPs to prescribe medications. It is important for each physician supervisor to determine what services he or she wishes his or her extenders to perform within the limit of the extenders' training and applicable state laws.

If your practice provides services in the areas in which physician extenders are capable of providing support, extenders may be a good option to handle the demand for more services.

Adding Physicians

Adding a new physician to your practice is the most costly option to handle the demand for patient services. However, if you have determined that adding a physician is the best option, you should be prepared to undertake a thorough analysis of your practice to determine the best and most cost-effective way to do so.

Benefits of Part-Time Physicians

The addition of a new, full-time physician to your practice has significant financial ramifications. There will be a need to generate additional revenue as soon as possible to prevent a reduction in compensation for the existing physician providers. One way to minimize this effect is to consider the use of part-time physicians.

Many practices that want to add an additional physician don't immediately need a full-time physician. Usually the growth in demand is such that a part-time person can handle the additional load at first. If this is the case, consider hiring a part-time physician. Depending on your local market, there may be opportunities to hire physicians who want to work only a few days a week. If so, this can be a cost-effective way to solve your needs.

Before making the decision to go with a part-time physician, you will need to check into the limitations this may create and other financial considerations such as the availability of medical malpractice insurance for part-timers.

Paying for an Additional Physician

The cost of hiring the new physician can be significant in terms of the cash commitment your practice must make. In addition to the actual hiring expenses, there may be a shortfall in revenue for a period of time. Volume of new patient visits for the physician usually grows slowly, as will the revenue from those visits and services. If you have guaranteed a minimum or base salary for the new physician, there may be a negative cash flow for a period of time.

Alternate or additional sources of revenue should be explored. For example, you may wish to consider providing services as a medical director for various entities such as nursing homes, public health or other clinics, or local emergency medical services (EMS) departments. Either you or the new physician may provide services in these areas. You may also consider adding services such as house calls or calls to nursing homes or assisted living facilities (ALFs). This alternative source of revenue is applicable for physician extenders as well.

Under certain circumstances, a local hospital may assist in providing funds for recruitment or salary guarantees. Recent law changes have limited these opportunities, but it is still worth contacting the administrators at the hospitals for which you provide care. They may also have opportunities for paid medical director positions, which can help offset the cost of a new physician.

Containing Costs in Recruitment

Once the decision to hire a physician or physician extender has been made, the process of recruitment must begin. There are several ways to approach recruitment. You must determine which method is the best for your practice and then attempt to contain the costs involved in the process.

Professional Recruiters

There are many professional recruiters available to help in the process of recruiting and hiring a new physician or physician extender. While the fees quoted may seem high, hiring a professional recruiter still may be the least expensive route to take. To determine the true cost, you must look at the services provided by the recruiting firms and what the value is to your practice.

First, you should consider the services of several recruiting firms before determining which one you will use. You should carefully review the services they will provide and the fees they will charge. Only after this process is complete will you be able to determine the best choice. In determining the firms to contact you may wish to inquire with the professional societies or organizations of which you are a member to see if they endorse one or more recruiting firms. You may also ask other physicians in your area if they have used the services of recruitment firms. Once you have made a list, contact each firm and ask for a list of their services and the fees they charge.

Most firms will provide resumes of potential physicians or extenders who meet your requirements. The firms may also arrange for the candidate to visit your practice. In addition, the firms may assist the candidate with others services, such as gathering information about your area or town that will be needed for him or her to determine whether he or she is interested in your practice opportunity. The recruiter may also assist you with employment information or documents and other services that are necessary.

Many recruiting firms have established lists of interested physicians or physician extenders who are actively looking for new positions. As a result, recruiting firms may be able to fill your position very quickly. In addition, some recruiters do a good job of screening potential candidates. This will eliminate unqualified candidates or those who would not be a match for your practice, greatly reducing the time you might spend on interviewing.

Some recruiting firms even "guarantee" hires to the extent that if the new hire does not work out within a specified period of time they will recruit a replacement at no additional cost.

However, there are recruitment firms in business that do not provide many of these services or those that have a poor track record in assisting practices but still charge high fees. Therefore, you must carefully qualify the firms you are considering by asking other clients they have served or check with the endorsing societies for their recommendations and insight. Carefully ask questions of the firms' representatives and get all promises in writing.

Recruiting by Yourself

If you choose to recruit a new physician or physician extender yourself, there are a number of areas of potential cost containment you can consider. Before you begin to recruit, you will need to assess your needs and the opportunities available in your area.

After you have determined the qualifications you want in a new physician or physician extender, you must determine the best method to begin the recruitment. You will first need to generate a list of potential candidates. How you do this is a product of the availability of candidates in your area and the method to reach them. Some methods to reach potential candidates are more expensive than others.

Advertising   Advertising for candidates is a good method to generate a list of potential associates, but advertising costs can be great. One of the most expensive ways to advertise is usually by placing an ad in a large-circulation newspaper. Depending on your area, this may or may not be effective. If you are in a large metropolitan area with a good supply of the type of provider you are looking for, this may work well. But you should also consider other places to advertise.

Specialty newspapers, such as local medical business newspapers, provide a more targeted approach and cost far less per potential contact. Newsletters, which list classified opportunities for the providers you are searching for, can also be effective and cost far less. Check with you professional societies at the local, state, and national level to see whether they provide these services. (See the following sidebar for sources of physician extenders.)

Sources of PAs, NPs, and Midwives

Following is a list of sources of physician extenders that may be helpful in your search for PAs and NPs, as well as midwives.

Allied Healthcare Search
Phone: 800 262-4194
Web site: www.alliednet.com

American College of Nurse Midwives
Phone: 202 728-9860
Web site: www.midwife.org

Midwife Alliance of North America
Phone: 888 923-6262
Web site: www.mana.org

American Academy of Physician Assistants
Phone: 703 836-2272
Web site: www.aapa.org

American Academy of Nurse Practitioners
Phone: 512 442-4262
Web site: www.aanp.org

When placing an advertisement, be sure to list the important requirements you may have for the position so that you can screen unqualified candidates, saving you unnecessary time and money.

Other Methods of Finding Candidates   There are other ways to find candidates to fill your new position that are cost-effective and may save you time. Start by letting the local hospitals know that you are looking for a new associate. Most hospitals receive letters of inquiry from physicians hoping to move to that area. This can be a ready supply of recruits.

You should also talk with the local medical society executives and let them know you are looking. They also receive letters from physicians interested in the area. In addition, they may know of local physicians who are interested in merging their practice with others.

Consider talking with your medical school or residency program as well as any other medical teaching program in your geographic area for potential physicians. These programs not only will know who is available but can give you accurate information as to the physicians' skills and competence. This can be your best source of qualified candidates.

If you are looking for a physician extender, contact the various state societies for the extenders and find out whether they publish a newsletter or operate a job-find service for their members. These, too, can be a cost-effective means of finding candidates who are qualified and licensed in your state.

Once you have found candidates to consider, it is time to begin the process of qualifying the candidates and interviewing the most promising. You will have to do most of the screening services provided by the recruiting firms in the process of finding the right associate, so be methodical and careful and utilize the right help in the search. Doing it yourself can be a big cost-saver and can find the right person for your practice.

Retaining Your Practitioners

The cost of retaining your physicians and physician extenders is far less than the cost of hiring new staff. Make sure you have policies and practices in place that will help retain these individuals, starting with fair and well-thought-out employment agreements, followed by reasonable compensation packages. In addition, make sure you provide the opportunity for effective communication between the professionals in your practice and growth and educational opportunities.

If you address these needs, you will be able to better retain the key providers in your practice and, in the long run, contain the cost associated with professional recruitment and retention.

Chapter 7

Optimal Organization Structures

H ow physicians choose to organize and operate their practices can have a significant effect on cost containment. While the preceding chapters in this book have dealt with specific areas of operation that can impact a practice's costs, the structure within which the practice functions has not yet been discussed.

This chapter looks at a number of ways a practice can be structured to help contain costs. The analysis of the various alternatives is therefore limited to their effect on *cost*—no attempt will be made to analyze other effects of such structures that may have significant impact on the practice and physicians. Before considering any change in a practice's structure, all potential effects must be reviewed and analyzed. For example, in *Practice Affiliation: Forming or Joining a Partnership or Group Practice,*[1] Barbara Hoagland indicates that physicians consider both philosophical and practical considerations when choosing the structure of their practices. Often the philosophical considerations outweigh the practical in the decision-making process. Because these philosophical issues can affect so much of the decision, they should be given careful attention.

Changes in the practice of medicine brought on by managed care have also created an impact on the organizational structure of the physician practice. The demand for greater information on the amount and quality of care has put pressure on the cost side of the equation. Making the decision to participate or not participate in a health plan requires the ability to gather data on your practice's costs. Deciding to offer new services or add new diagnostic tests and procedures, again, requires the data for proper analysis. The right organization can help provide this information in a cost-effective way.

The ability to operate a practice in a cost-effective manner is greatly determined by the availability of qualified individuals and effectiveness with which they are used. It is necessary to keep the number of employees to a minimum because of the cost in retaining them. At the same time, this seems counter to the need to have enough qualified help. How you meet these needs will have an effect on how you organize your practice.

The optimal organizational structure, therefore, is a combination of the acceptable philosophy and the most efficient organization.

Solo versus Group Practice

The decision to practice in a group setting or on your own has many considerations.

It is clear that the number of physicians choosing to practice in a solo setting is declining. Between 1991 and 1995 the number of physicians in solo practice declined by 22%, from a total of 34.1% in 1991 to 26.5% in 1995.[2] At least part of the reason for this trend is the need for physicians to practice more efficiently. Studies have shown that large groups are more efficient than solo practices.[3] Such efficiency is determined not only by practice costs but also by physician productivity.

Staff Costs

Demands on practices to provide more data to third-party payors along with increased administrative duties have put pressure on practices to add more administrative personnel. In addition to quantity, the quality of staff required has been elevated. Dealing with complex regulations for billing and managed care operational requirements have forced practices to hire a higher level of employee.

The cost of staff has been a big factor in the lower efficiency of solo practices. The ability to share new staff with multiple physicians does not exist. Hiring part-time staff with specific skills such as managed care billing and collections is more difficult than hiring full-time staff. In addition, it is cost-prohibitive to hire qualified practice managers in a solo practice.

Conversely, group practices are able to hire specialists in various areas of practice operation because of the practice's larger revenue base. And the cost of a well-trained practice manager is within the financial ability of a larger group practice.

Well-trained and experienced practice managers, whether they are called office managers, practice administrators, or chief operating officers, can have a significant impact on practice costs. The implementation of the various strategies listed in this book requires an individual with good training and understanding in the

The number of clinical staff necessary to run the practice generally increases in the same proportion as physician providers, so there tends not to be a cost benefit in this area as the number of providers grows.

operations of a medical practice. Such an individual is compensated at a higher level than are most general office workers. However, such a person should be able to save the practice an amount far in excess of his or her salary and benefit costs. Still, it is hard to justify such a highly paid position in a solo practice. Clearly, staff costs can be held to a more reasonable level in a group practice and become more reasonable as the group increases in size.

Forming a Group Practice

There are two ways to approach the formation of a group practice. If you are currently in a solo practice, you can recruit new physicians to join your practice, thus forming a group. The alternative is to merge your solo practice into an existing group practice. While the two methods require different legal steps and documents, the end result is the same.

Before you form or join a group, it is important to clearly define the reasons you have for taking this step. Those reasons can help identify your goals and give you the basis for a business plan necessary to achieve success. In addition, if one of your purposes in forming or joining a group practice is to help reduce or contain costs, you should make a list of the areas in which you hope to achieve the cost savings.

Once you have identified the areas of potential cost savings, you must carefully analyze each to determine how you plan to reduce costs. Too often practices think they will realize savings before they restructure, only to find out later that the changes actually led to increased costs.

Personnel Questions

As one of the greatest areas of cost for a practice is in personnel, staffing is the logical place to start an analysis. Generally it is wise to divide the personnel into *clinical* and *administrative* to begin this analysis.

Questions to be asked and answered include:

- Can you share staff with an additional practitioner?

- Which staff will have to be added to the new group practice?

- Can existing staff be let go?

Be realistic in your analysis and include your practice administrator in the process. Also, remember to add the other costs of personnel into your calculations, such as employee taxes and benefits.

General Overhead

Another area to analyze is the effect on general overhead in the formation of the group. Will more office space be needed? How much new equipment will have to be purchased? What will the effect be on utilities and insurance? Carefully make these calculations.

Variable Costs

Finally, consider the effect the group formation will have on the variable cost of the practice, such as office supplies, medical supplies, and other supplies. It is also important to factor in any potential savings you may receive by being able to order larger quantities of these supplies.

Sharing Office Overhead

Another alternative to forming a group practice or adding a practitioner to your practice is an arrangement to share office overhead with an independent physician. Such arrangements provide many of the cost savings of adding practitioners but with limited responsibility and organization dynamics.

Under this type of an arrangement, a practice will provide a workplace for an independent physician and provide some or all of the support services needed for an agreed-upon fee. Such arrangements can reduce the practice's overhead expenses for each physician and still enable independence of the physicians.

A carefully worded agreement, which specifically lists the services provided and the expectations of the parties to the agreement, is critical. And, as with any affiliation, a careful evaluation of the physician who will share the space must be undertaken to make sure the practice styles are compatible.

Understanding the Effect of Economies of Scale

It is common to hear that by getting bigger you will benefit from economies of scale. Basically this statement means that you will use less resources to produce a greater volume of goods or services. This maxim works in some cases but not in all cases.

Don't assume that bigger is always more cost-effective. You must first under-stand the nature of expenses and how they are affected by volume of services to determine whether an increase in service volume will realize cost bene-fits. In *Medical Practice Accounting & Finance: A Practical Guide for Physicians, Dentists, and Other Medical Practitioners*, Rose Marie Bukics and Donald Chambers explain the different characteristics of fixed, variable, and semivariable costs[4]:

Costs that are *fixed* for a given practice will not change with an increase in volume and therefore can be considered to be contributory to an economy of scale. Such costs as rent and depreciation don't change with an increase of patients or the addition of a new practitioner, assuming you have adequate space in the office and don't buy new, expensive equipment. However, if it is necessary to move the office to allow for more space, a new fixed cost must be calculated.

Costs that vary in direct proportion with the volume of services provided are referred to as *variable costs*. Good examples of variable costs in a practice are medical supplies and office forms. If the volume of patients increases by 20%, these costs will also go up by 20%. As a result, variable costs will not be a factor in calculating any economies of scale. It is important to remember that, should the volume of some of these expenses increase, such as supplies, it may be possible to reduce your per-unit cost by receiving a volume discount in purchasing.

Many costs fall under the category of *semivariable* or *step variable*. These types of costs will remain fixed for a range of volume increase or decrease and then increase to a higher fixed level over the next range of volume increase or decrease. Personnel costs generally fall under this classification of costs. A practice may be able to see five or six more patients during a day without the need to hire more staff. But at some point the volume increase will require that you hire a new staff member. At that point the cost jumps up to a new level for personnel costs. Your ability to calculate the points at which these types of costs will increase is important to calculating the potential of obtaining cost efficiencies as your practice increases volume.

Additional Methods to Contain Costs Organizationally

In an effort to optimize the organizational structure of a practice, several other options exist that can lead to cost containment. These options are generally referred to as *outside affiliation options*.

Solo practices that do not want to consider expansion into group practices or groups that do not want to expand may wish to consider the following options to help meet the demands of the current medical marketplace without expanding their office overhead significantly. As was discussed earlier, one of the most significant areas of cost pressure is in the area of personnel costs. Practices are seeing the need to provide more sophisticated billing and practice management systems, the need to hire seasoned practice managers, and the need to deal with more and more complicated regulations, while the pressure to reduce or contain costs is the greatest it has ever been. Rather than trying to meet these demands internally within the practice, several options exist that can address these needs at a lower cost.

Practices can affiliate with outside organizations that provide many of the services needed without the up-front investment. One such type of affiliation is with a management services organization (MSO). In *Integrating the Practice of Medicine: A Decision Maker's Guide to Organizing and Managing Physician Services*, Paul DeMuro defines an MSO as "an organization that provides services to physicians and physician group as well as others."[5]

MSOs have increased in number in the past few years. Many were started as a result of failed physician practice management companies. As practices were purchased and run by these practice management companies, the individual practices lost the ability to provide certain services within the practice. When the companies failed and either sold or gave back the practices to the physicians, the practices were not equipped to perform the tasks. Companies were formed that were able to provide these services, and in many cases, these companies could do so at a lower cost than the individual practices could.

Some of the services provided by MSOs include billing and collections, group purchasing, managed care contracting services, utilization management, and management information services. Because of their size, many MSOs are able to contract for greater discounts in supplies and other services used by the physician practices. The MSOs are also able to keep up with changes in regulations and billing requirements more easily. In addition, some of the challenges of personnel administration are eliminated for the physicians.

As with all alternatives that may lead to cost savings, the services and costs involved with the affiliation with an MSO must be carefully reviewed. A cost analysis of the services provided and the cost to the practice must be undertaken to determine whether you are truly saving money under this alternative. It is also important to check references for the MSO to see if the practices they provide services to are happy with the arrangement.

Other affiliations such as with independent practice associations (IPAs) and physician hospital organizations (PHOs) may provide additional alternatives. Such affiliations will probably provide fewer services than an MSO but will likely cost less too. Areas of strength for IPAs and PHOs generally lie in the areas of managed care plan operations and control and information systems. In some cases the IPAs or PHOs may contract with an outside MSO to provide some or all of these services.

As with the MSO, you must carefully evaluate the IPA or PHO before you consider affiliation. Some widely discussed failures of these organizations have reinforced the necessity to approach such a decision with care and good information. Still, there are good and effective IPAs and PHOs in business, and they do offer an alternative to providing in-house services in some areas.

However you choose to organize your practice, remember that there are potential cost savings to be realized with the right alternatives. Carefully evaluate these options and develop the optimal organization structure for your practice.

Endnotes

1. Hoagland B. *Practice Affiliation: Forming or Joining a Partnership or Group Practice.* Chicago, IL: American Medical Association; 1990.

2. *Socioeconomic Monitoring System Survey*, 1991-1995. Chicago, IL: American Medical Association.

3. Emmons DW, Kletke P. Physician practice size, 1991-1995. In: Connors RB, ed. *Integrating the Practice of Medicine: A Decision Maker's Guide to Organizing and Managing Physician Services.* American Hospital Publishing; 1997.

4. Bukics RM, Chambers DR. *Medical Practice Accounting & Finance: A Practical Guide for Physicians, Dentists, and Other Medical Practitioners.* New York, NY: Probus Publishing; 1995.

5. DeMuro PR. Evolution of management services organizations. In: Connors RB, ed. *Integrating the Practice of Medicine: A Decision Maker's Guide to Organizing and Managing Physician Services.* American Hospital Publishing; 1997.

Afterword

Managing a medical practice can be an arduous task if the physician is not properly organized. The key to successfully operating a medical practice efficiently and cost-effectively is twofold: First, the physician must have a carefully thought-out plan to approach the task. Second, the physician must understand the concepts and methodologies that have been presented in this text and must be willing to utilize these tools in making changes.

It is common for a physician to read a text such as this and decide that his or her practice could benefit from making changes that will aid in managing costs. Unfortunately, many physicians begin the process but fail to bring it to fruition because the process entails some steps that require extra work or skill sets that he or she does not possess, or creates a potentially unpleasant situation for a short period of time.

Physicians desiring to modify practice operations to enhance cost saving and improve efficiency must commit to working through the necessary processes. Once the changes have been planned, implemented, and monitored, the practice will begin to experience positive improvements. Many of these improved operational efficiencies will occur gradually and a reduction in costs will be noted over time.

It is important to remember that in analyzing the results of the changes made to the practice that the physician look at trends over a period of time from 3 to 6 months. Reviewing changes on a weekly or monthly basis will not allow for peaks and valleys in performance. Therefore, it is important to study trends over an extended time period and fine-tune the various parts of the practice as needed.

The practice that sees the benefit in improving operations, analyzes the practice's needs, properly plans changes to be made, and utilizes an implementation plan will be successful in attaining its goals. Remember, an efficiently and effectively managed practice will have many of the following benefits:

- The practice will more readily adapt to industry changes in the future.

- Expenses will decrease and workflow will be more efficient.

- The practice stress level will decrease and the staff will be happier and more productive.

The ability to operate an efficient and cost-effective practice rests solely with the physician. If you are willing to make the commitment, you will reap the benefit.

Appendix A

Leading Health Care IT Companies

Following is a listing of the top 25 health care system vendors in the marketplace today, as ranked in the June 2000 issue of *Healthcare Informatics*.

Rank 2000	1999	Company Name and Location	Primary Business
1	1	McKessonHBOC Alpharetta, GA 800 891-8601 www.hboc.com	Enterprise-wide patient care, clinical, financial, and strategic management software solutions, and networking technologies, e-commerce, outsourcing, and other services; 5% of the annual revenue is attributed to health care IT.
2	3	EDS Plano, TX 800 566-9337 www.eds.com	Information and e-business technologies to private and public health care enterprises; 7% of the annual revenue is attributed to health care IT.
3	2	SMS Corp. Malvern, PA 610 219-6300 www.smed.com	Health information systems and services, including ASP delivery, outsourcing, e-commerce, managed Internet, and enterprise systems management; 100% of the annual revenue is attributed to health care IT.
4		3Com Corp. Santa Clara, CA 800 638-3266 www.3com.com	Voice and data networking; 14% of the annual revenue is attributed to health care IT.
5	6	CSC El Segundo, CA 800 272-4799 www.csc.com	E-business strategies and technologies, management consulting and integration, application software, IT, and business process outsourcing; 7% of the annual revenue is attributed to healthcare IT.
6		Varian Medical Systems Palo Alto, CA 800 544-4636 www.varian.com	Radiotherapy systems for treating cancer; 10% of the annual revenue is attributed to health care IT.
7	4	SAIC San Diego, CA 800 544-7242 www.saic.com	Integration services, including HIPAA, e-business, telecom, desktop, network, and program management; 9% of the annual revenue is attributed to health care IT.

Rank		Company Name and Location	Primary Business
2000	**1999**		
8	5	NDC Health Information Services Atlanta, GA www.ndchealthcenter.com	Products and services to pharmacies, hospitals, physicians, payors, and other health care providers; 100% of the annual revenue is attributed to health care IT.
9	8	IDX Systems Corp. Burlington, VT. 802 862-1022 www.idx.com	Develops and implements IS.
10	7	Cerner Corp. Kansas City, MO 816 221-1024 www.cerner.com	Clinical and management IS; 100% of the annual revenue is attributed to health care IT.
11	9	MedQuist, Inc. Marlton, NJ 800 233-3030 www.medquist.com	Electronic medical transcription and health care information management solutions; 100% of the annual revenue is attributed to health care IT.
12	29	Per-Se Technologies, Inc. Atlanta, GA 877 737-3773 www.per-se.com	Integrated business management services, application software, and Internet-enabled connectivity for providers; 100% of the annual revenue is attributed to health care IT.
13	11	Medic Computer Systems, Inc. Raleigh, NC 800 334-8534 www.medic.com	Clinical, e-commerce, and Internet solutions to practices and hospitals; 100% of the company's total revenue is attributed to health care IT.
14	16	Ingenix, Inc. Eden Prarie, MN 888 445-8745 www.ingenix.com	Clinical and cost management solutions for payors, providers, employers, pharmaceutical manufacturers, government agencies, and others; 100% of the annual revenue is attributed to health care IT.
15	18	Eclipsys Corp. Delray Beach, FL 561 2431440 www.eclipsys.com	End-to-end IS for health care clinical, financial, and satisfaction outcomes; 100% of the annual revenue is attributed to health care IT.
16	10	Data General Westboro, Mass. 508 898-5000 www.dg.com/healthcare	High-technology enterprise solutions; 17% of the annual revenue is attributed to health care IT.
17	19	Quadra Med. Corp. San Rafael, CA 800 871-0633 www.quadramed.com	Web-enabled, secure solutions that link hospitals to their diverse constituents; 100% of the annual revenue is attributed to health care IT.
18	13	Medical Information Technology, Inc. (MEDITECH) Westwood, MA 781 821-3000 www.meditech.com	Solutions for integrated delivery systems, long-term care facilities, and other health care organizations; 100% of the annual revenue is attributed to health care IT.
19	14	First Consulting Group Long Beach, CA 800 345-0957 www.fcg.com	Information-based consulting, integration, and management services to health care, pharmaceutical, and other life sciences organizations; 90% of the annual revenue is attributed to health care IT.

Rank		Company Name and Location	Primary Business
2000	1999		
20		ACS Dallas, TX 800 845-5530 www.acs-inc.com	Technology, application, and business process products and services for health care financing and delivery organizations; 11% of the annual revenue is attributed to health care IT.
21	28	Medical Manager Health System Tampa, FL 800 222-7701 www.medicalmanager.com	Integrated health care automation solutions; 100% of the annual revenue is attributed to health care IT.
22	12	Lanier Worldwide, Inc. Atlanta, GA 800 708-7088 www.lanier.com	Document management solutions and services; 15% of the annual revenue is attributed to health care IT.
23	33	InfoCure Corp. Atlanta, GA 800 343-3279 www.infocure.com	Products automate practices in targeted medical specialties; 100% of the annual revenue is attributed to health care IT.
24	22	Oracle Corp. Redwood Shores, CA 800 672-2531 www.oracle.com	Supplier of software for information management; 2% of the annual revenue is attributed to health care IT.
25	15	PeopleSoft, Inc. Pleasanton, CA 925 225-3000 www.peoplesoft.com	Designs, develops, markets, and supports a family of enterprise e-business applications and Internet-based application software products.

Healthcare Informatics: The Business of Healthcare Information Technology. June 2000.

Appendix B

Physician Practice Management System Selection Evaluation

Following is a sample evaluation form to use when selecting a physician practice management system for your practice.

Vendor Script and Evaluation Criteria	Available	Not Available	Excellent (E), Good (G), Satisfactory (S), Unsatisfactory (US), Does Not Apply (DNA)	Comments
Patient Registration				
Enterprise-wide patient number and registration				
Ability to perform registration for another site				
Comprehensive patient registration and editing functionality				
Copy of demographic information from screen, patient guarantor				
System edits for duplicates, etc.				
Adequate space for addresses, information, free text				
Audit trail on registrations and changes				
System information: • HMO/PPO subscriber number • Cash required alert				
User-defined information for insurance coverage screen				

Vendor Script and Evaluation Criteria	Available	Not Available	Excellent (E), Good (G), Satisfactory (S), Unsatisfactory (US), Does Not Apply (DNA)	Comments
Automatic benefits and eligibility check through online links				
Patient chart/charge ticket, labels, user-defined forms				
15+ user-defined patient notes				
Provide for preregistration to capture demo data prior to visit				
Ad hoc reporting graphs				
Provide batch interface to accept registration data from other systems				
Ability to set up and retrieve of HMO/PPO eligibility data				
Registration of recurring/series patient				
Multiple fee schedules				
Ability to time stamp for patient check-in				
Discuss process of online eligibility reporting and review				
Discuss how the membership database works				
Patient surveillance module and statistics reporting				
Discuss system ability to "flag" collection accounts				
Discuss referral tracking				
Discuss patient "look-up" (inquiry)				
Provider Maintenance				
Track provider credentials				
Contract renewal dates and warn of expiring contracts				
Historical tracking and statistics				
Check patient assignments from registration				
Link referral providers to individual or network contracted payment arrangements				
Track hospital affiliations with specific privileges				
Charge Posting				
Detailed and summary service reports				

Vendor Script and Evaluation Criteria	Available	Not Available	Excellent (E), Good (G), Satisfactory (S), Unsatisfactory (US), Does Not Apply (DNA)	Comments
Alerts for duplicate charge posting				
Audit checks within the system (eg, reasonableness check, number, % amount, etc.)				
Ability to look up patient by name or number				
Accommodate fourth-and fifth-digit editing of diagnosis code				
Default diagnosis				
Demonstrate audit trail or charge transactions				
Ability to override information (price, procedure, etc.)				
Support multiple fee structures				
Calculation of contractual terms				
Daily and monthly audit reporting				
Denial explanation fields				
Ability to generate ad hoc reports/graphs				
Ability to post to specific charges				
Billing				
Discuss how payor demographics are established/edited				
Discuss claim data requirements, edit checks				
Electronic billing and reporting				
Automated balance billing to secondary payors				
Contract management system and reports				
Discuss handling of capitated contracts				
Ability to perform centralized and decentralized billings				
User-defined reporting				
Discuss audit trails				
Review billing cycle options				
Ad hoc reports and graphs				

Vendor Script and Evaluation Criteria	Available	Not Available	Excellent (E), Good (G), Satisfactory (S), Unsatisfactory (US), Does Not Apply (DNA)	Comments
Claims Processing/Adjudication				
Use of authorized services is linked to claims and payments and how IBNR (incurred but not reported) is documented as claim is paid on the referral				
Autopayment by diagnosis				
Provide sample of IBNR exposure reporting				
Claims processing/adjudication				
User-defined managed care reporting				
Claims Management				
Automated user-defined claims correspondence				
Online subscriber, eligibility, and benefit verification through online link				
Electronic transmission of claims through ANSI standards				
User-defined unlimited edits with claims management and reporting				
Online claim level notes				
Upload or error correction by carrier				
Electronic transmission of claims through ANSI standards				
Electronic funds transfer				
Ad hoc reports and graphs				
Full transmission history				
Generation of copayments and deductibles				
Referral/Authorization				
Link multiple authorizations for patient				
Tight integration with interaction with claims processing				
Ability to document referral management process				
Ability to document authorization process by payor				
Ability to generate referral authorization report/letter				

Vendor Script and Evaluation Criteria	Available	Not Available	Excellent (E), Good (G), Satisfactory (S), Unsatisfactory (US), Does Not Apply (DNA)	Comments
Ability to track number of visits against number of referrals				
Automatically calculate estimated liability based on contracts/authorized services				
Provide IBNR (incurred but not reported) reports				
Provide estimated versus actual liability reports for closed authorizations				
Generate referral and authorization forms. User-defined?				
Detect duplicate authorizations				
Support online unlimited user-defined notes				
Ad hoc reports and graphs				
User-defined reporting				
Collections				
Collection follow-up system				
Online worklists and reports				
Enterprise-wide collections				
What coding schemes are available for comments				
User-defined setup of comments for letters, bills, statements				
Review statement setup and parameters (financial class, age balance, patient type, practice, groups)				
Autodialing capability				
Payment plans and reporting				
Combining of accounts and audit checks				
Monitoring tools and reports				
User-defined bad debt processing				
Automatic letter follow-up routine? Can they be free text?				
Standard and free text messages				
Free text and standard comments use				
Guarantor versus patient billing				

Vendor Script and Evaluation Criteria	Available	Not Available	Excellent (E), Good (G), Satisfactory (S), Unsatisfactory (US), Does Not Apply (DNA)	Comments
User-defined statements				
Ability to send to outside agency user-defined parameters.				
Ability to perform centralized and decentralized collections				
Collector performance tracking				
Ad hoc reporting and graphic capabilities				
Ability to place statement on hold				
Archiving/Security				
User-defined archiving of accounts				
Review security				
Scheduling System				
Integrated scheduling of physicians, rooms, equipment and other resources				
Ability to review schedule on weekly, daily, and monthly basis				
Capture of referring and primary care physician information				
Capture of visit duration information/tracking information				
Additional unlimited information or comments at scheduling				
Outstanding balances.				
Collector notes/alerts at scheduling				
Cancellation of all or part of physician's schedule with automatic search for new scheduling time slot				
Multiple office/facility scheduling with conflicts				
Ability to double or triple book				
Automatic sequence of appointments by test/procedure				
Ability to schedule more than one resource per time and room				

Vendor Script and Evaluation Criteria	Available	Not Available	Excellent (E), Good (G), Satisfactory (S), Unsatisfactory (US), Does Not Apply (DNA)	Comments
Interface to hospital admissions or scheduling for enterprise scheduling				
Ad hoc reporting				
Allow overbooking and overlaps by specific time periods				
Search by patient, day of week, time of day, duration				
Block out times easily, including recurring slots				
Automatic update of all system on appointments				
Bring daily, weekly appointment list				
Ability to report reason for visit				
Multiple physicians on one screen				
Automatically alerts medical records for chart pull				
Ability to monitor patients from check-in to discharge with statistics				
Schedule physicians for at least 6 months				
Ability to produce ad hoc reports				
Ability to define unlimited schedule definitions				
Medical Records				
Computerized patient record				
Electronic signature				
Ability to define treatment protocols with standard templates by specific type				
Customization of patient charts				
Bar coding chart management				
Laptops, palmtops, or portable laptops for clinical documentation that provide real-time update via radio-frequency (RF)				
Problem lists with staging of illnesses				
Acuity weighting tools				
Ease of tools/flowsheets				
Allergy list available				

Vendor Script and Evaluation Criteria	Available	Not Available	Excellent (E), Good (G), Satisfactory (S), Unsatisfactory (US), Does Not Apply (DNA)	Comments
User-defined/free text progress notes				
Automatic tracking of medication history				
Online formulary by payor				
Ability to print prescriptions				
Drug, food, and allergy interactions				
Laboratory/numerical flowsheet form				
Ability to print images, documents into record				
Ability to interface transcription into electronic chart				
Online user-defined correspondence				
Centralized or decentralized chart management				
Ad hoc reports and graphs				
Patient Services Management				
Entry and tracking of patient service issues				
Integrated correspondence/ word processing				
Patient satisfaction monitoring and reporting				
Support of user-defined parameters for tracking and resolution of issues				
Historical database of issues and related information				
User-defined form letters				
User-defined patient service parameters				
Patient Survey generation and reporting/statistics				
Ad hoc reports and graphs				
Wait time tracking				
Payment Posting				
Electronic remittance				
Review payment/system balancing protocols				
Ability to post by name, ID#, SS#, INS#				
Ability to edit				
Ad hoc reports and graphs				

Vendor Script and Evaluation Criteria	Available	Not Available	Excellent (E), Good (G), Satisfactory (S), Unsatisfactory (US), Does Not Apply (DNA)	Comments
Report Generation				
Review report production capabilities				
Discuss system flexibility				
Ease of Use				
Menu-driven with logical structure plain language				
Window-oriented screen displays				
Error messages in plain English				
Speed				
Time to register a new patient (goal: 1 minute)				
Patient access time (goal: 2 seconds)				
Menu searching time (goal: 2 seconds)				
Hardware and Software				
Review purging and archiving				
Operations Management				
Discuss backup protocol				
Describe daily, weekly, monthly processing				
Review the systems management process				
Discuss the company's application support and education				
Reliability				
Backup performed within the program				
Built-in reindexing				
Files editing available				
Vendor is well established				
Source code in escrow				
Program author(s) available				
Telephone support available				
Modem support available				
Discuss downtime and disaster recovery				
Technical Support				
Discuss hardware configuration				
Discuss devices supported by system				

Vendor Script and Evaluation Criteria	Available	Not Available	Excellent (E), Good (G), Satisfactory (S), Unsatisfactory (US), Does Not Apply (DNA)	Comments
Does system support use of PCs as terminals or network devices?				
Is system compatible with area-wide network?				
Credentials				
Track provider credentials				
Contract renewal dates and expiration warnings				
Historical tracking and statistical data				
Check patient assignments from registration				
Electronically link referral providers to individual or network contracted payment arrangements				
Track hospital affiliations with specific privileges				
A/R				
How payor demographics are established/edited				
Claim data requirements, edit checks				
Electronic billing and reporting				
Automated balance billing to secondary payors				
Contract management system and reports				
Discuss handling of capitated contracts				
Ability to perform centralized and decentralized billings				
User-defined reporting				
Discuss audit trails				
Review billing cycle options				
Ad hoc reports and graphs				
Electronic remittance				

Selected Organizations Certifying Office Professionals

The American Health Information Management Association (AHIMA)

In 1991 the American Medical Record Association (AMRA) changed its name to the American Health Information Management Association (AHIMA). It is responsible for establishing excellence standards in health information management. The Web site, www.ahima.org, is a great resource to learn more about the organization and its activities.

Recently, the AHIMA conducted a benchmarking survey and it found that 39% of its members work in physician group practices, 26% work in hospitals/integrated delivery, 21% are employed in ambulatory care/surgical centers, and 14% are employed in managed care. The AHIMA has a membership of over 40,000 professionals who work throughout the health care industry.

Some of the human resources needed for physician practices include the following:

- **Registered Health Information Administrator (RHIA) (formerly Registered Record Administration)**

  RHIAs are skilled in the collection and analysis of patient data. In a recent membership survey, AHIMA found that more than half of the RHIA respondents were directors, managers, or consultants, with nearly 31% serving as health information directors. Minimum requirement is a bachelor's degree.

- **Registered Health Information Technician (RHIT) (formerly Accredited Record Technician)**

  RHITs are health information technicians who ensure the quality of medical records by verifying their completeness, accuracy, and proper entry into computer systems. RHITs often specialize in coding diagnoses and procedures in patient records for reimbursement and research. In AHIMA's recent membership survey, the majority of RHIT respondents held job titles in either of the following categories: coding/technician or manager/supervisor.

  Minimum requirement is an associate degree from an accredited Health Information Technology (HIT) program.

- **Certified Coding Specialist (CCS)**

  CCSs are professionals skilled in clarifying medical data from patient records, generally in the hospital setting. To perform this task, CCSs must possess experience in the ICD-9-CM coding system and the surgery section within the CPT® medical code coding system.

  Minimum requirements are high school diploma and 3 years' on-the-job coding experience and education.

- **Certified Coding Specialist–Physician-Based (CCS-P)**

  The CCS-P is a coding practitioner with expertise in physician-based settings such as physician offices, group practices, multispecialty clinics, or specialty centers. The coding practitioner reviews patients' records and assigns numeric codes for each diagnosis and procedure. CCS-Ps possess knowledge of the CPT® medical code coding system and familiarity with ICD-9-CM and HCPCS level II coding systems.

  Minimum requirements are a high school diploma and 3 years' coding experience and education.

The AHIMA has a wonderful Web site that has a current list of community colleges and undergraduate degree programs by state. In addition, there is complete information on requirements, seminars, and testing sites for certification, as well as continuing education.

The Professional Association of Health Care Office Managers (PAHCOM)

PAHCOM was founded in 1988 to provide a support system to the managers of physician office practices. It has over 3000 members. For members of PAHCOM who are actively involved in medical office management, there is a certification process. The following information is obtained from PAHCOM's Web site (www.pahcom.com) or interviews with its staff.

- **Certified Medical Managers (CMMs)**

  To qualify for certification, medical office managers must:

  1. Be actively employed as a health care office manager for a minimum of 3 years.

  2. Successfully complete at least 12 college or university credits. (There is an extensive experience recognition option wherein the educational credit requirement is reduced by one credit hour for every year of experience the candidate has above the 3-year minimum. For example, a candidate with 15 or more years of experience would not need any formal education credits.)

  3. Be recognized as a health care office manager by both peers and employer(s).

  Candidates for the CMM must take a two-part written examination. Part 1 is composed of 160 multiple-choice questions about relevant management knowledge in health care. Some of the covered areas are as follows: billing and collections, coding analysis, communication, conflict management, financial planning, human resources, patient education, practice marketing, practice structure, risk management, third-party reimbursement, and time management.

  Part 2 requires the candidate to provide comprehensive responses to two of three case studies that depict complex problems in managing a health care practice. PAHCOM publishes the *PAHCOM Management Guidebook*, which serves as the main text for development of the certification exam.

  PAHCOM also has a requirement of 24 hours of continuing education units (CEUs) every 2 years. This helps ensure CMMs are current about changes in the health care practice environment.

American Academy of Professional Coders (AAPC)

The mission of the AAPC incorporates the establishment and maintenance of professional, ethical, and educational standards for all parties concerned with procedures in coding medical information. Much of the information here is obtained from interviews with the AAPC and from their Web site, www.aapcnatl.org.

As of June 2000, there were 16,500 members of the AAPC. The AAPC certifies coders in the following two areas:

- **Certified Professional Coder (CPC)**

  The CPC is primarily for physician practice coders. The test is open book and it consists of a 5-hour exam with 150 questions (multiple choice and true or false). Individuals are tested on medical terminology, human anatomy, evaluation and management services, surgery coding, medicine section coding, CPT® medical code, and ICD-9-CM Volumes 1 and 2, to name a few of the areas. There is a continuing education program that CPCs are encouraged to attend to maintain their certification.

- **Certified Professional Coder–Hospital (CPC-H)**

  The CPC-H is primarily for physician services coding in a hospital. The format of the exam is similar to the CPC. However, questions include the format of the UB-92 claim form, medicate guidelines, and reimbursement issues. There is also a continuing education program that CPC-Hs are encouraged to attend to maintain their certification.

  An example of a recent job from the AAPC *Coding EdgeCareer Bulletin* (May-June 2000) reads as follows:

  Consultant/Coding Specialist

  Candidate will lead medical group business office turnaround and compliance assessments for independent groups and integrated delivery systems throughout the country. Will also conduct reimbursement analysis and provide CPT-4/ICD-9 coding training for physicians. Must have hands-on management experience, full knowledge of coding and billing procedures, and superior communication skills. Five years health-care experience. BA required. CPC desired. Travel. Benefits.

Index